Residential Care

Your Role in the Health Care Team

- A Guide to Common Health Problems
- Working with Doctors
- Medications, Step-by-Step

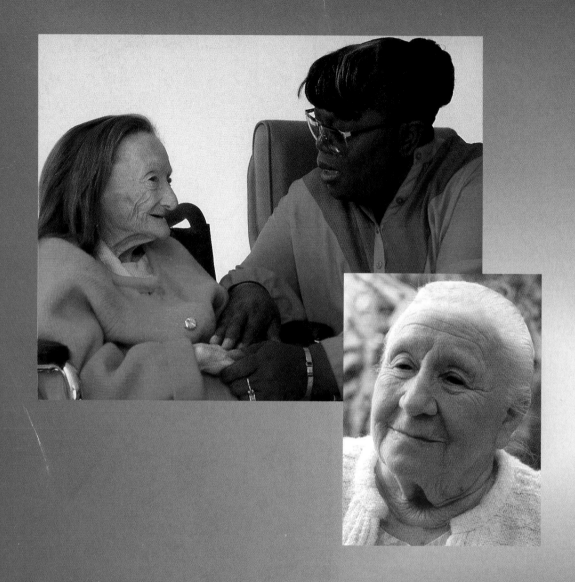

- A Guide to Common Health Problems
- Working with Doctors
- Medications, Step-by-Step

Residential Care
Your Role in the Health Care Team

Harvey K. Swenson RPh
Vice President, Regional Director of Consulting
Pharmacy Corporation of America

Jay S. Luxenberg MD
Director, Fellowship Program in Geriatric Medicine
Medical Training Director,
UCSF/Mt. Zion Center on Aging

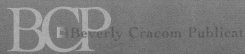
BCP Beverly Cracom Publications

St. Louis, MO   Wilton, CT   Pasadena, CA

A joint venture between Beverly Foundation and Cracom Publishing, Inc.

BCP
■Beverly Cracom Publications

Publisher & Editorial Director: Barbara Ellen Norwitz
Senior Editor: Donna Frassetto
Development Editor: Marny Johnson
Production Editor: Chris Cook
Design: Bill Drone, Mary Siener
Production: Mary Siener
Manufacturing: Michael Kemper

Photography: Lightworks Photography & Design, Annapolis, MD
George D. Dodson

Notice: The authors and publisher of this volume have attempted to offer easy-to-use information and assessment tools that are currently accepted and used by professionals in related fields. Nevertheless, changes in the health care delivery and reimbursement systems as well as new pharmaceuticals and medical technology will alter the application of some concepts and techniques presented in this text. The publisher and authors disclaim any liability, loss, injury, or damage incurred as a consequence, directly or indirectly, of the use and application of any of the contents of this volume.

Library of Congress Cataloging-in-Publication Data
Residential Care: Your Role in the Health Care Team
Harvey K. Swenson, RPh
Jay S. Luxenberg, MD

Includes bibliographical refences and index.
ISBN: 1-886657-06-8
1. Nursing home care I. Title.
RC954.3.S93 1996   95-48453
362.1'6—dc20   CIP

Printed in the United States of America

10 9 8 7 6 5 4 3 2 1

Preface

There has always been a need for caregivers to assist frail elderly or sick people whose families could not provide the necessary care. As modern sanitation and improved nutrition and health care have made living to an advanced age an expectation for most of us rather than the exception, the need for additional help for the oldest and most infirm has grown dramatically. Today's family is often scattered and younger generations are likely to be committed to school or workplace. Fortunately, along with the increasing need for nonfamily care of the elderly, a variety of care settings has developed that allows us to hope for a safe and healthy living environment if we become physically or mentally needy as we age.

The common and disabling illnesses of old age—such as arthritis, dementia, and diabetes—are not cured, but rather are managed over the long term with medications, appliances, and day-to-day care. In these situations, an older person often needs help with daily tasks. The housework that used to be routine now becomes difficult or even impossible. Using a bathtub becomes a nightmare, and a single slip can shatter a hip or break an arm. Shopping and preparing meals may be too difficult, and malnutrition or even starvation can occur. Mental confusion can put one at risk of being cheated or abused, and unpaid bills can lead to embarrassing or even dangerous problems.

One way to manage is to move into a facility where others share the need for help, to decrease costs while receiving more care for the money available. This is where *residential care—the care that you are providing*—enters into the picture. Yet moving from home into an institution, even one as friendly as a small neighborhood facility, is a difficult and often frightening experience. Most of us hope that we never need such care, but statistics indicate a likelihood that we will at some time in our lives. By giving up a certain amount of control over our day-to-day life, we expect to be safe in a clean, healthy environment.

This book will help you to provide such a safe and healthy environment in your residential care facility. Section 1 examines types of residents and your responsibilities to them. Section 2 explores how to plan their care, including when to contact the resident's doctor. Section 3 discusses common health problems. Your residents are likely to have various illnesses and to be taking several medications, so Section 4 is devoted to understanding medications.

Your responsibilities regarding the administration of medications will vary with facility policy and state laws. Section 4's Medication Quick Reference chart identifies families of medications, brand and generic names, common uses, important side-effects, and directions for use. The best techniques of medication storage and record keeping are also reviewed.

One difficult task in providing excellent residential care is deciding when a medical condition or behavior problem makes the resident unsafe in your facility. Although no book can answer all such questions, the information about the care needs of common medical problems can be very helpful when you need to evaluate a current or potential resident.

Many facilities require staff to administer medications and perform minor treatments. The information in this book will guide you and your staff in these tasks. You may find it useful to share this book with your staff and to keep it in a handy location—difficult questions can pop up at the oddest times in residential care! We hope that you will find the illustrations and tables useful, and that the format makes finding important information easy.

Harvey K. Swenson
Jay S. Luxenberg

Dedication

To my wife Jane whose unfailing support was absolutely essential, to the board and care managers who generously offered their time and assistance, and to the many elderly persons who taught me so much about their needs and who made me understand their value to us all.

Harvey K. Swenson, RPh

I would like to thank my family for their support and encouragement throughout the process of developing this book.

Jay S. Luxenberg, MD

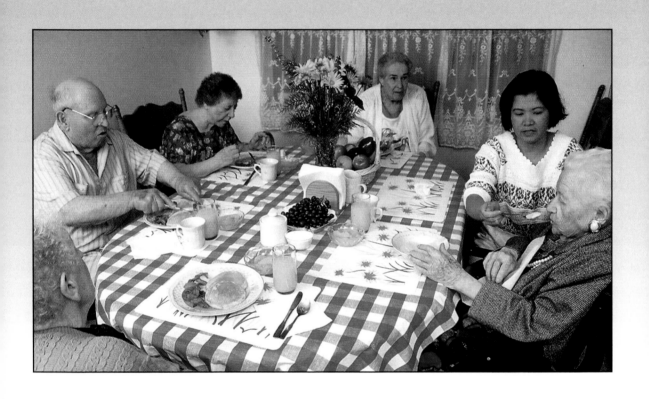

Table of Contents

SECTION 1
THE RESIDENTIAL CARE ALTERNATIVE   3

   A Growing Need   3

   Role of the Residential Care Facility   4

   Types of Residents   6

   Specializing in the Elderly   8

   Responsibilities and Limitations   9

   You and Your Staff   11

   Resources   18

SECTION 2
HOW TO PLAN CARE   25

   Understanding Your Residents' Needs   25

   The Initial Evaluation   26

   Admission Record   27

   Care Plans   30

   Keeping Records Current   32

   When A Resident Needs More Care Than You Can Provide   39

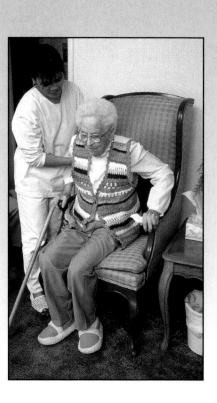

SECTION 3
COMMON HEALTH PROBLEMS   43

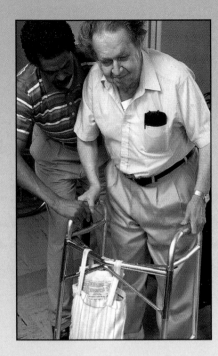

Abdominal Pain   44

Angina and Coronary Artery Disease   51

Ankle Swelling   56

Arthritis   60

Bladder Problems   65

Broken Bones   72

Cancer   77

Congestive Heart Failure   83

Constipation   87

Cough   92

Dementia   97

Diabetes   102

Diarrhea   108

Falls   112

Fever and Chills   116

Headache   120

Heart Attack   124

High Blood Pressure   129

Kidney Failure   133

Movement Disorders and Seizures   137

Musce or Bone Pain   142

Nausea and Vomiting   146

Poor Sleep   150

Pressure Ulcers   154

Psychiatric Disorders 160

Rash 165

Sensory Impairments 170

Shortness of Breath 174

Stroke 178

Weakness or Numbness 183

SECTION 4
UNDERSTANDING MEDICATIONS 189

Your Role 189

How Medications Work 190

Labeling 198

Guidelines and Techniques 201

Common Problems 225

Medication Quick
Reference 234

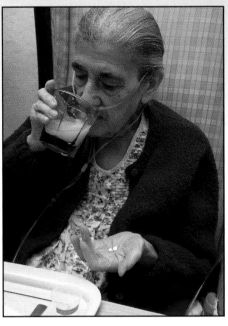

APPENDICES 277

Appendix 1: Residential Care
Facility Health Resources 277

Appendix 2: Measurement Equivalents 282

Appendix 3: Common Medical
Abbreviations 283

Appendix 4: Drug References 285

Appendix 5: Sample Residential
Care Forms 289

Glossary 297

Index 303

Residential Care

Your Role in the Health Care Team

- A Guide to Common Health Problems
- Working with Doctors
- Medications, Step-by-Step

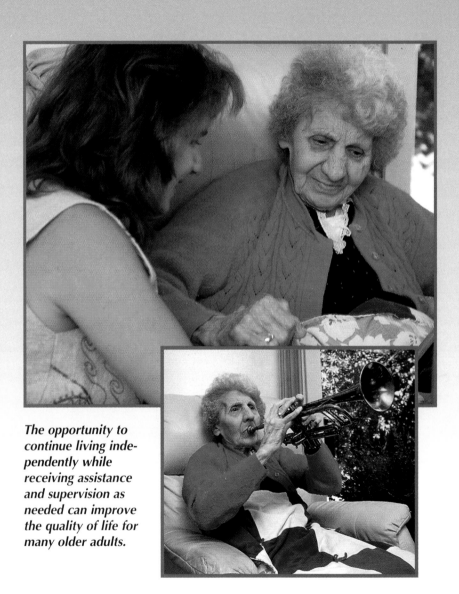

The opportunity to continue living independently while receiving assistance and supervision as needed can improve the quality of life for many older adults.

1

The Residential Care Alternative

A GROWING NEED

The idea of homes for the elderly originated long ago, but historically, it has been the family who took care of an elderly parent or parents who could no longer care for themselves. Households commonly included three generations, and the youngest and oldest, by turns, provided care for each other. Major social changes and scientific advancements have served to change these traditions, with several factors being especially important.

- As more wives joined the workforce, there was no one at home to provide care needed during the day.

- Increased divorce rates and the resulting increase in single-parent families left the elderly without care or assistance during at least part of each day.

- Families became more mobile, moving from place to place, often in search of jobs, making it difficult for the extended family to stay together.

- Finally, medical advances have resulted in more of us living to an older age. The so-called frail elderly or very old (85 and older) represent the most rapidly growing segment of the elderly population. This group is far more likely to need some

▣ OTHER TERMS USED FOR RCFs

- Assisted living center
- Adult foster home
- Board and care home
- Care home
- Domiciliary care home
- Family home
- Home for the aging
- Home for elderly
- Rest home
- Sheltered living home

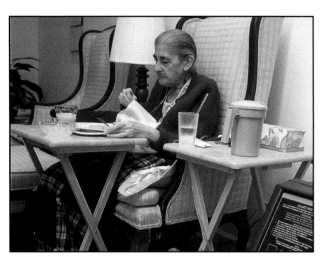

Individuals who are 85 years of age and older are the fastest growing segment of the elderly population.

sort of assistance in performing routine activities of daily living and to require medical care than is someone 20 years younger at 65, the age that used to be considered "old."

Two issues have strengthened the position of residential care facilities (RCFs): the desire of elderly persons to stay at home for as long as possible and the need to control constantly rising health care costs. Residential care facilities, which provide a home-like environment, with relatively low costs and opportunities for social and environmental stimulation, help to meet these objectives. In addition, living in a supervised environment helps the resident avoid debilitating and costly health problems such as dehydration, malnutrition, adverse drug reactions, falls, and fractures. So, although residential care facilities have been around for a long time, their numbers are increasing and their importance in our society is growing.

ROLE OF THE RESIDENTIAL CARE FACILITY

Residential care facilities vary considerably in size as well as in services they offer. Some may be as small as 3 to 6 residents, but many

WHAT RCFs ARE

- Homes for people who need assistance with activities of daily living, often including some degree of personal or health care

WHAT RCFs ARE NOT

- Nursing facilities or intermediate care facilities

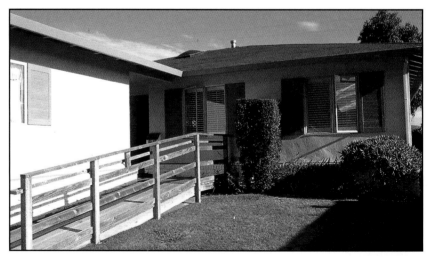

Residential care facilities are not defined by size and many are private homes that have been modified to meet the needs of a small group of residents.

care for well over 100. Although residents rate social services and activities highest among their priorities, the steadily increasing number of the "very old" has resulted in more emphasis on a facility's ability to meet daily health needs and provide assistance with routine daily activities. It is no longer unusual to find facilities that offer services very similar to those provided by skilled or intermediate care nursing facilities. Some RCFs have separate facilities that provide licensed nursing care on the same campus. Within the same facility, some residents may be self-sufficient, requiring only minimal assistance with cleaning, laundry, and shopping. Other residents may need a level of assistance that is much higher. In between are many levels of care and services, based on resident needs and the resources of the facility.

The RCF challenge, then, is to help residents maintain as much physical and mental function and independence as possible in a non-medical setting.

Although RCF charges vary widely depending on location, types of services, and the quality and surroundings in which the services are provided, RCFs represent an important and relatively inexpensive alternative in the care of the elderly. RCFs are nearly always substantially less expensive than nursing facility care. Some RCFs can even be less expensive than congregate living or home care when the cost of outside services (home health aides, Meals-on-Wheels, taxis to events, etc.) are factored in.

Especially to the small operator, there can be real advantages beyond the opportunity to profit from the use of one's home and basic cooking and care skills. For many, there is a value in the companionship of their residents, many of whom become more like friends or family than residents. For younger operators, there

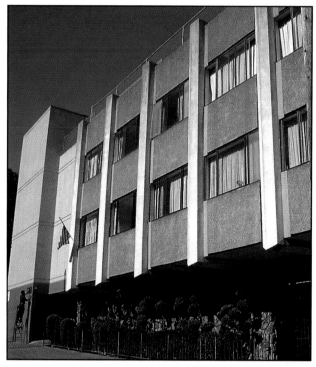

Larger residential care facilities share the goal of helping residents remain as independent as possible.

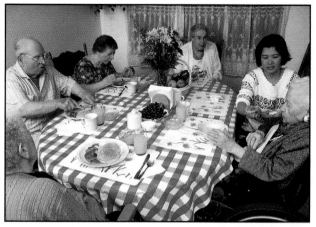

The needs of residents will vary, but most consider the company of other residents a primary benefit.

is a chance to involve the entire family in the enterprise, providing not only financial rewards for children, but a much better understanding of the elderly than most of their friends will ever have. Finally, there are the rewards of being able to work at home and the chance to work for oneself that many small RCF owners enjoy.

TYPES OF RESIDENTS

Although the primary focus in this book is elderly residents, we realize that many facilities provide services to a mixture of elderly and non-elderly residents. Specific characteristics of these groups are discussed below.

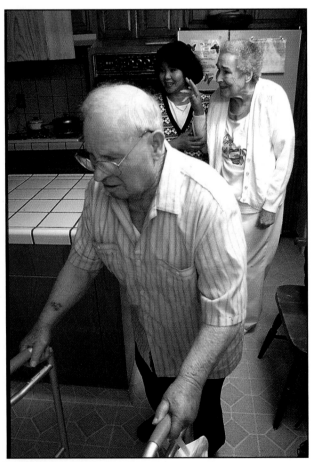

Assistance with meals and activities of daily living, as well as help with medications or trips to the doctor, may be all a resident needs.

The Elderly

The term *elderly* is generally taken to mean persons over 65 years of age. However, we all know people who are very vigorous and healthy at that age, and others who are younger but are quite frail.

Many elderly persons who cannot or choose not to live at home anymore simply need a congregate living arrangement that offers homemaker services, meal options (dining room or self-preparation of meals), and travel assistance for shopping trips, doctor's office visits, and the like. They live alone, or with a spouse or roommate. In spite of their relative independence, these people may have one or more chronic medical conditions, and they often need increased levels of care and assistance as they grow older and lose some physical or mental function, or both. Some RCFs, which are primarily congregate living facilities, have special units within the facility where extra care is provided, sometimes by licensed or registered nurses.

Other RCFs specialize in caring for residents with chronic physical or mental conditions whose only other option would be a skilled nursing or intermediate care facility.

The Mentally Disabled

Over the past 20 to 30 years, changes in drug therapy and the philosophy of care for the mentally disabled has led to an increased demand for non-medical sheltered environments for persons with chronic mental illness. The most common form of mental disability in the elderly is dementia, but there are also elderly persons with long-standing psychiatric conditions such as schizophrenia who need RCF services. These residents provide extra challenges for the RCF manager and caregivers:

- These residents are just as likely to have the same physical ailments as other elderly residents.
- They are more likely to resist care efforts.
- Their medications often must be managed for them.

RCF managers who have a high proportion of residents over 80 years of age should expect about half of their residents to develop irreversible and progressive dementia. They should understand that dementia is a primary cause of serious accidents in and around the home.

The Physically Disabled

As with mental disability, some degree of physical disability is to be expected in nearly all older persons. These disabilities may eventually cause the resident to have to be transferred to a higher level of care. However, some RCFs do accept younger residents with chronic physical disabilities along with elderly residents. We all know the benefits we get from interaction with those younger than us— we learn about new things that we probably would have ignored, and we stay a little sharper. People talk about children keeping them young. Although not children, younger residents can be a positive influence in an RCF by giving older persons a different perspective that can help to prevent residents from withdrawal and a narrowing of interests. On the other hand, these younger residents can also present special problems. Besides the

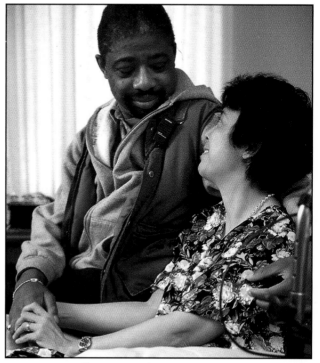

Some RCFs allow married couples with chronic physical disabilities to live together.

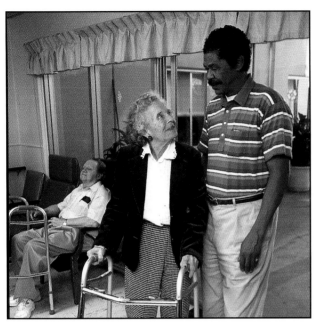

Whether an older person lives at home or in a residential care facility he or she is equally likely to suffer from a chronic medical problem or require some help during recovery from a sudden illness or period of hospitalization.

obvious concern for their ability to perform activities of daily living and mix well with the rest of the home's residents, many of these residents will have progressive disabilities that will require both careful monitoring and, possibly, transfer to another level of care.

SPECIALIZING IN THE ELDERLY

Elderly persons in a residential care facility are usually not significantly different from elderly persons in the general population in regard to basic health problems, but they vary significantly in the degree of disability resulting from those diseases or in their resources or ability to care for themselves. For example, older persons living at home and those in RCFs, as a group, are about equally likely to suffer from chronic diseases such as heart disease or high blood pressure (hypertension). However, the RCF resident is likely to be older by an average of five or six years, is far more likely to have had a disabling condition such as stroke, and is unable to perform essential tasks, called "activities of daily living" (ADLs) without assistance. (ADLs include eating, sleeping, bathing, toileting, and similar routine tasks.) Because of the effects of chronic disease, people living in RCFs are far more likely to suffer from at least occasional urinary incontinence, more likely to suffer from the effects of dementia and depression, more likely to fall, and more likely to need help with everything from showering to taking medications.

Case Examples

The individuals in the following three cases would all benefit from a residential care facility that specializes in the elderly.

A 78-year-old woman is having increasing difficulty in cooking, cleaning, keeping her clothes clean, and going out shopping, as well as having trouble remembering to take her medications properly. She could try to get someone on a part-time or live-in basis to do all of these things, but finding competent, trustworthy, and reliable helpers is complicated and can be very expensive. On the other hand, she may decide to go to an RCF or other assisted living environment and let someone else take care of everything while she gets the benefit of interaction with others her age. With assistance, she is also more likely to take her medications properly and thereby decrease the risk of reactions that cause so many elderly persons to be hospitalized because of falls, dehydration, or other serious medication side effects.

An elderly diabetic man has recently had an amputation of one leg below the knee. After surgery and a brief hospitalization, he stayed at a rehabilitation nursing facility until he no longer needed skilled nursing care. The RCF environment represents a chance to continue to learn to use his prosthesis, or artificial limb, and to recover enough physically to be able to return home.

A stroke victim has either had only a mild stroke or has recovered substantially in a nursing facility from a more severe stroke. Placement in an RCF would provide simple assistance with recovery efforts, which might include assistance with walking and range-of-motion exercises (perhaps in concert with a visiting therapist), swallowing exercises, and the like.

RESPONSIBILITIES AND LIMITATIONS

Legal Definitions

Because health care itself is heavily regulated in most states, legal limitations on resident services vary. For example, some facilities are able to provide care for persons who have had strokes who can barely communicate their needs and require almost total assistance with ADLs. RCFs that do not specialize in complex care usually find it necessary to provide some assistance with the administration of medications for some residents, assistance with bathing or other ADLs, and help in managing medical problems. This latter assistance may take many forms, from assisting residents in making appointments and visiting doctors, to taking direct action to help residents deal with minor ailments or problems, to

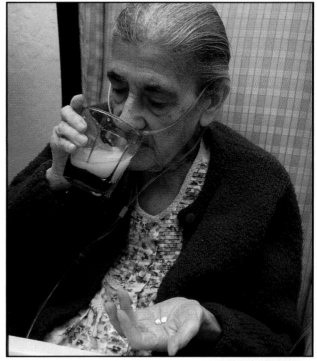

Home health technology permits a higher level of care to be received in the residential setting than in the past.

A wide variety of safety and home health devices can help improve the resident's sense of security and physical well-being.

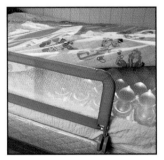

Air mattress and bed rail

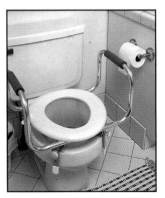

Elevated toilet seat and grab bars

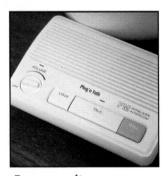

Room monitor

reporting observed or reported symptoms or behaviors to a resident's doctor or family member. RCF operators and managers should carefully evaluate their capabilities to determine the kind of residents for whom they can provide care. Those wishing to provide a higher level of care should be prepared to invest in the necessary training.

RCF operators who want to provide these higher-level care services need to be sure that they are doing so within the law. This can be complicated, since there are no federal standards, and there are wide variations in the state and local rules that apply. If a particular act, such as helping a resident administer insulin, is not addressed in RCF regulations, practice acts for nurses could conceivably prohibit laypersons from providing the care. RCF associations can ask government agencies about the legality of certain kinds of care without putting a specific facility at risk by identifying it.

An evaluation of the responsibilities of RCF operators and managers begins with any requirements your state has for facilities like yours. These standards will establish minimum guidelines, and they may also place limits on what you may do for your residents.

However, whatever state laws and regulations apply to your facility, your primary responsibility is to be personally qualified for the level of assistance and care your residents need and to be able to assist in transfers when a resident requires a different care setting.

Safety and Security

One of your basic responsibilities is the safety and security of your residents. Usually, state or local licensing laws require minimum standards for all types of care facilities. Even if yours is not a licensed care facility, potential residents and their families will have safety and security uppermost in their minds as they search for a satisfactory care facility. Common sense is important. For example, smoke alarms, railings, grab bars (especially in bathrooms), and non-skid bathtubs and showers should be routinely available in any facility that cares for elderly people. Additional measures are important, such as limiting access to kitchen stoves or fireplaces when you have residents who are confused or otherwise mentally impaired, as well as understanding signs of confusion or other mental disability that may affect the judgment of your residents. Also, you must take the necessary, additional precautions for residents with specific needs, such as making sure those with limited ambulation (walking) ability do not have to manage steps or other obstacles. Some modification of the living environment or training in new skills may be required for you and your staff.

■ TYPES OF ASSISTANCE

This book cannot give you nursing or medical skills, but it will help you to make the day-to-day decisions that will help ensure the comfort, safety, and appropriate level of assistance for your residents. Examples of the types of assistance you may need to provide include:

- Activities of daily living (ADLs) such as bathing, grooming, dressing, and errands

- Special diets, feeding, and nutrition

- Closer supervision for temporary illness

- Medication purchases, safe storage, and administration

- Contacting doctors' offices to arrange medical care

- Communicating with doctors and other health professionals regarding specific elements of care

- Transportation for social activities, errands, and medical care

- Networking with community resources

- Helping arrange for skilled nursing or intermediate care as needed

- Helping resident return home when possible

- Observing residents carefully enough to communicate with doctors and family and know when to call

- Basic first aid, such as helping with bandages

- Physical and psychological support for specific resident needs

YOU AND YOUR STAFF

RCF staffing needs, or the number of residents per caregiver, will vary greatly depending on the physical layout of the facility and resident needs. More staff may be needed during the daytime hours than at night.

Most new residents will come from their own homes, and even the most pleasant of surroundings cannot replace a person's own home. Satisfaction with your facility, and even the health of your residents, depends on good food, the companionship of amiable peers, and, perhaps most importantly, the attitude, competence, and availability of your staff. Although this book is not intended to be a training manual, the importance of proper caregiver selection, orientation, and training deserves special emphasis.

■ WHAT YOU CANNOT DO

- Provide care that is limited by law to doctors, nurses, or other licensed health care workers unless they are employed by you and can legally provide those services in your facility

- Provide any care that you are not competent to provide

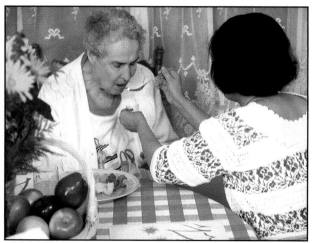

The attitudes and availability of your staff are important to the well being and comfort of your residents.

Attitudes

Whether working with elderly persons or others needing care, certain characteristics in caregivers are essential. Besides the expected traits of honesty, reliability, flexibility, and a willingness to learn and work hard that every employer looks for, RCFs must focus on other attributes as well. Chief among these is a genuine affection for or interest in your residents. Not everyone is comfortable around elderly persons, and many potential caregivers who would work well in another environment simply may not have the ability to relate well to your residents. The same can be said for others who may work well with older people but not with the mentally ill, developmentally disabled, small children, or teenagers.

It is important to determine before hiring possible negative attitudes caregiver applicants may have about the kind of residents for whom you care. Some applicants may be desperate for employment and seek jobs that they know will be especially difficult for them. Unfortunately, this tends to work out poorly for your residents, who will quickly realize that the caregiver is not comfortable with them. This, in turn, may result in residents not requesting care when they should or developing a general feeling of mistrust.

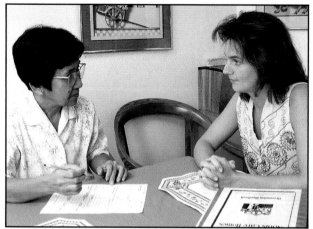

Qualifications of your staff include, but are not limited to, experience in health care.

Rules of Conduct

Some states have taken official notice, through fingerprint screens for criminal records, of another especially important caregiver qualification—honesty. As with anyone involved in personal care, RCF caregivers have access to personal items that are prized possessions of your residents, regardless of their worth to others. Coupled with a tendency for some elderly people to become suspicious of the motives and actions of others (sometimes with good cause), the importance of honesty, together with very well-defined rules of conduct for caregivers, cannot be overstated.

Other important caregiver qualifications include:

- Language skills appropriate to your residents
- Physical strength (for those involved in providing direct physical assistance with activities such as bathing)
- Reasonably good health (Elderly immune systems, especially among those over 80 years of age, are not as good in resisting colds and other infections.)

Important *personal* caregiver characteristics include:

- Honesty, trustworthiness
- An honest interest in and appreciation of your residents
- Patience
- Intelligence, especially for those performing complex tasks
- Cleanliness
- Recognition of the importance of their work

Finding the Right Employees

The search for caregivers with these qualifications may best start with people who have already demonstrated the necessary skills, knowledge, and experience that will help you ensure your residents the best possible care. A few states have begun to define minimum skill standards for RCF caregivers, similar to what has been done for certified nursing assistants (CNAs) in nursing facilities. In fact, nursing-facility trained CNAs and those providing home care services offer skills and knowledge that are ideal for RCFs as well. Of course, CNAs trained in or for nursing facilities will need to understand that RCFs are different from other care settings and that resident capabilities will differ substantially from those of nursing facility residents.

Other persons who tend to work well and learn quickly in RCFs are those who have had experience caring for loved ones with the same needs as your residents. When someone has met the needs of an elderly mother, father, aunt, uncle, or friend, they not only know what is involved, but they are likely to know whether it is something they *like* to do as well.

For caregivers such as licensed or registered nurses or certified home health aides, or even, in some states, registered, licensed, or certified RCF aides, state government will have already done some of the work for you. Usually these people have been fingerprinted and at least some check of criminal background has been made. Even so, you will need to check references yourself and interview applicants

▧ WHERE TO LOOK FOR CAREGIVERS

- Certified nursing assistants
- Home health aides
- Those who have taken care of relatives or friends at home
- Relatives and friends who are capable and willing
- Agencies providing services off-site, such as nursing facilities (for housekeeping, laundry, or dietary personnel; direct caregivers will be CNAs), adult day health care centers and other RCFs
- Outside agencies providing on-site services, such as home health agencies and hospice agencies

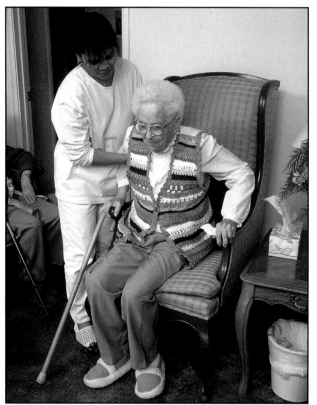

Some skills may need to be individualized for the needs of your residents, however, many skills are basic and universal to almost any care setting.

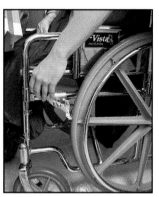 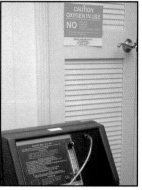

In addition to basic care activities, staff training should also include specific precautions and skills that apply to the health needs of your residents, for example, how to use wheelchairs and walkers properly, and precautions for in-house use of oxygen.

carefully. Your employees will be working with people who are at special risk for theft and deception, and a license or certificate is not enough. For those for whom there is no government background check, your check of references is even more important.

Employee Orientation and Training

Successful businesses and organizations know the value of effective orientation and ongoing training for their employees. This holds true even for small RCFs. Careful selection of new employees can be largely negated by careless orientation and a lack of commitment to continued training.

Effective orientation starts with well-defined policies and procedures, prefer-ably written, that provide consistent guid-ance and set performance standards. Resources such as this book can be used both to increase caregivers' knowledge and to provide a quick reference for spe-cific care issues that are not included in policies and procedures.

For example, it is important to know your own limitations and those of your staff. It is equally important to develop training opportunities that will help you and your staff learn and improve care skills. The more you know about your res-idents' health and the more you know of the needs you can satisfy within the frame-work of your state regulations, the more likely a resident is to feel comfortable and secure in your facility.

Figure 1–1, Caregiver Checklist, may help you identify services that you can pro-vide or may be able to improve on, based on the knowledge and experience of you and your staff and the physical limitations of your facility.

Caregivers need to be sensitive to the fact that residents, as adults, have certain rights in any care delivery system. The Patient's Bill of Rights shown in Figure 1–2 was developed by the American Hospital Association to formalize guidelines for health care professionals in the acute care setting. Your staff should also be familiar with these rights because their philosophical basis is applicable to every care setting.

Figure 1-1 **Caregiver Checklist**

- Ability to communicate verbally and in writing in the language of most residents
- Physical ability to assist residents with their needs
- Freedom from communicable diseases such as TB that could harm residents
- Certification as nursing assistant or home health aide or previous experience assisting persons with similar problems/disabilities to those found in your facility
- Basic knowledge of physical and mental limitations common in elderly, including risk of skin tear or breakdown, bowel and bladder control, hearing and visual impairment, dietary changes, and mobility limitations
- Acceptable standards of hygiene
- General knowledge of activities and social services needed by elderly persons
- Ability to assist with bathing, dressing, and feeding residents
- Ability to provide care to incontinent residents
- Proper care and use of various assistive devices such as walkers and wheelchairs
- Terminology and procedures for administering medications
- Knowledge of conditions and circumstances that require a doctor's attention
- Safe lifting techniques
- Prevention of falls and other accidents
- Fire safety precautions
- Proper response to medical emergencies
- Philosophy of care and limits on care in your facility
- Resident rights and an understanding of the nature and consequences of elder abuse
- Fire, earthquake, flood, and other disaster readiness

Figure 1-2 **AHA Policy A Patient's Bill of Rights**

Introduction

Effective health care requires collaboration between patients and physicians and other health care professionals. Open and honest communication, respect for personal and professional values, and sensitivity to differences are integral to optimal patient care. As the setting for the provision of health services, hospitals must provide a foundation for understanding and respecting the rights and responsibilities of patients, their families, physicians, and other caregivers. Hospitals must ensure a health care ethic that respects the role of patients in decision making about treatment choices and other aspects of their care. Hospitals must be sensitive to cultural, racial, linguistic, religious, age, gender, and other differences as well as the needs of persons with disabilities.

The American Hospital Association presents *A Patient's Bill of Rights* with the expectation that it will contribute to more effective patient care and be supported by the hospital on behalf of the institution, its medical staff, employees, and patients. The American Hospital Association encourages health care institutions to tailor this bill of rights to their patient community by translating and/or simplifying the language of this bill of rights as may be necessary to ensure that patients and their families understand their rights and responsibilities.

Bill of Rights*

1. The patient has the right to considerate and respectful care.

2. The patient has the right to and is encouraged to obtain from physicians and other direct caregivers relevant, current, and understandable information concerning diagnosis, treatment, and prognosis.

    Except in emergencies when the patient lacks decision-making capacity and the need for treatment is urgent, the patient is entitled to the opportunity to discuss and request information related to the specific procedures and/or treatments, the risks involved, the possible length of recuperation, and the medically reasonable alternatives and their accompanying risks and benefits.

    Patients have the right to know the identity of physicians, nurses, and others involved in their care, as well as when those involved are students, residents, or other trainees. The patient also has the right to know the immediate and long-term financial implications of treatment choices, insofar as they are known.

3. The patient has the right to make decisions about the plan of care prior to and during the course of treatment and to refuse a recommended treatment or plan of care to the extent permitted by law and hospital policy and to be informed of the medical consequences of this action. In case of such refusal, the patient is entitled to other appropriate care and services that the hospital provides or transfer to another hospital. The hospital should notify patients of any policy that might affect patient choice within the institution.

4. The patient has the right to have an advance directive (such as a living will, health care proxy, or durable power of attorney for health care) concerning treatment or designating a surrogate decision maker with the expectation that the hospital will honor the intent of that directive to the extent permitted by law and hospital policy.

    Health care institutions must advise patients of their rights under state law and hospital policy to make informed medical choices, ask if the patient has an advance directive, and include that information in patient records. The patient has the right to timely information about hospital policy that may limit its ability to implement fully a legally valid advance directive.

5. The patient has the right to every consideration of privacy. Case discussion, consultation, examination, and treatment should be conducted so as to protect each patient's privacy.

6. The patient has the right to expect that all communications and records pertaining to his/her care will be treated as confidential by the hospital, except in cases such as suspected abuse and public health hazards when reporting is permitted or required by law. The patient has the right to expect that the hospital will emphasize the confidentiality of this information when it releases it to any other parties entitled to review information in these records.

7. The patient has the right to review the records pertaining to his/her medical care and to have the information explained or interpreted as necessary, except when restricted by law.

8. The patient has the right to expect that, within its capacity and policies, a hospital will make reasonable response to the request of a patient for appropriate and medically indicated care and services. The hospital must provide evaluation, service, and/or referral as indicated by the urgency of the case. When medically appropriate and legally permissible, or when a patient has so requested, a patient may be transferred to another facility. The institution to which the patient is to be transferred must first have accepted the patient for transfer. The patient must also have the benefit of complete information and explanation concerning the need for, risks, benefits, and alternatives to such a transfer.

9. The patient has the right to ask and be informed of the existence of business relationships among the hospital, educational institutions, other health care providers, or payers that may influence the patient's treatment and care.

10. The patient has the right to consent to or decline to participate in proposed research studies or human experimentation affecting care and treatment or requiring direct patient involvement, and to have those studies fully explained prior to consent. A patient who declines to participate in research or experimentation is entitled to the most effective care that the hospital can otherwise provide.

11. The patient has the right to expect reasonable continuity of care when appropriate and to be informed by physicians and other caregivers of available and realistic patient care options when hospital care is no longer appropriate.

12. The patient has the right to be informed of hospital policies and practices that relate to patient care, treatment, and responsibilities. The patient has the right to be informed of available resources for resolving disputes, grievances, and conflicts, such as ethics committees, patient representatives, or other mechanisms available in the institution. The patient has the right to be informed of the hospital's charges for services and available payment methods.

The collaborative nature of health care requires that patients, or their families/surrogates, participate in their care. The effectiveness of care and patient satisfaction with the course of treatment depend, in part, on the patient fulfilling certain responsibilities. Patients are responsible for providing information about past illnesses, hospitalizations, medications, and other matters related to health status. To participate effectively in decision making, patients must be encouraged to take responsibility for requesting additional information or clarification about their health status or treatment when they do not fully understand information and instructions. Patients are also responsible for ensuring that the health care institution has a copy of their written advance directive if they have one. Patients are responsible for informing their physicians and other caregivers if they anticipate problems in following prescribed treatment.

Patients should also be aware of the hospital's obligation to be reasonably efficient and equitable in providing care to other patients and the community. The hospital's rules and regulations are designed to help the hospital meet this obligation. Patients and their families are responsible for making reasonable accommodations to the needs of the hospital, other patients, medical staff, and hospital employees. Patients are responsible for providing necessary information for insurance claims and for working with the hospital to make payment arrangements, when necessary.

A person's health depends on much more than health care services. Patients are responsible for recognizing the impact of their life-style on their personal health.

Conclusion

Hospitals have many functions to perform, including the enhancement of health status, health promotion, and the prevention and treatment of injury and disease; the immediate and ongoing care and rehabilitation of patients; the education of health professionals, patients, and the community; and research. All these activities must be conducted with an overriding concern for the values and dignity of patients.

These rights can be exercised on the patient's behalf by a designated surrogate or proxy decision maker if the patient lacks decision-making capacity, is legally incompetent, or is a minor. © 1992 by the American Hospital Association, 840 North Lake Shore Drive, Chicago IL 60611

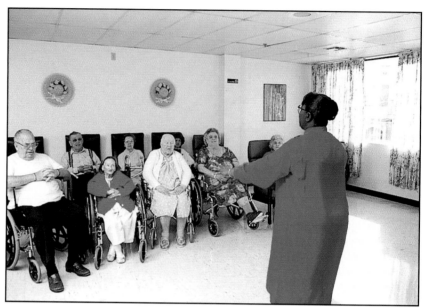

RCFs provide social activities for their residents.

RESOURCES

RCF managers need resources and special training to be effective. Many agencies and organizations are available to help provide these services, as well as to help broaden the range of services you can make available to your residents.

Except when family members can assist, or outside agencies are used for skilled nursing services, RCF direct care responsibilities, including assistance with ADLs and medications, must be met by the facility staff. Larger RCFs are usually better able to provide the social and activity services that are so important to the elderly, from simple in-house activities like bingo, to excursions for health care, shopping, fairs, and sporting events, to complex social services assistance. Smaller facilities may not have the resources for many of these services.

Licensing

There are nearly as many unlicensed RCFs in the United States as there are licensed facilities. Federal involvement in RCFs has been limited to the Keys amendment to a 1976 Social Security Act, which requires states to set and enforce standards for facilities where significant numbers of Social Security Insurance (SSI) recipients reside and to penalize those living in non-approved residences. Since the penalty provision has never been enforced, this law has not had a major impact on RCF standards of care. In the past several years Congress has shown the same kind of interest in residential care that it did in nursing homes prior to major changes in federal nursing home laws and regulations in 1974 and 1987. Some individuals in the Health Care Financing Administration (HCFA) are currently searching for ways to regulate RCFs via social security or Medicaid.

Interest at the federal level stems in part from the fact that state regulations vary greatly and, at least in some states, are viewed as ineffective. There is also concern that, just as nursing facility populations are sicker and older than in years past, some residential facilities are providing a higher level of care than before. That same reason—a need for a higher level of care—has prompted some states to consider statutory and regulatory change for existing licensed facilities and to propose actions to force unlicensed facilities to apply for licenses.

What this means to unlicensed facilities is that they should become familiar with state requirements for licensure, regardless of whether they intend to apply voluntarily for licensure. In some cases, state requirements may be a useful resource in providing care for residents. Each state, and some local jurisdictions, has regulations for facilities that provide care services to their residents. Enforcement of state laws and regulations is usually the responsibility of the state health department, department of social services, or department of aging. Some county-sized local jurisdictions enforce both local and state regulations for at least some licensed facilities. If you call or write to the agency most directly responsible for facilities of your type, the agency will either provide you with the necessary regulations or direct you to the appropriate legal codes.

Advocacy Programs

There are government agencies, usually located in a city or county health department or in a separate department of aging, that serve as advocates for elderly or disabled persons. In some cases they may provide consultative assistance to residential care facilities as well as to RCF residents. However, in most cases, unfortunately, government agencies act primarily in an enforcement role, and so are of limited value as resources to assist in providing services to your residents. Ombudsman programs may be helpful in some cases, although their primary focus is usually on advocating for individuals rather than facilities.

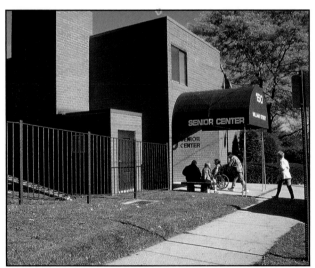

Residents can gain significant benefits from interaction with others and trips to other sites such as a community senior center where activities can provide physical, social and intellectual stimulation.

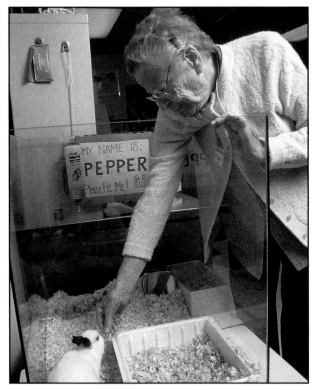

Adult day care can provide a variety of stimulating activities.

Community Services and Agencies

Most communities have senior activities programs, if not social services, usually through non-profit agencies or city or county government units like parks and recreation departments. These may offer nothing more than a chance to meet with other seniors for talk, games, or other recreation. This is a significant benefit to those in small RCFs, but many senior programs provide the kind of structured programs that some elderly persons require. Individuals receiving public assistance may already benefit from the social services assistance of a case worker. Social services for those residents without family support are more difficult to find. Local clearinghouse agencies are set up by counties or non-profit groups to provide information about services available to elderly persons.

Adult Day Care and Home Health Care

Health care services are provided by adult day health care centers, where older persons can get physical therapy, occupational therapy, speech therapy, and activities designed to maintain range of motion and other physical capabilities. Sadly, there are relatively few of these agencies, and even fewer in small communities. These agencies may give first priority to older clients living at home, because the original purpose of these centers was to allow people in need of services to remain in their homes. In most cases, adult day health care centers are state or county licensed, and contacting state or county agencies is one way to locate them. They can also be found through the primary county agency for the aging.

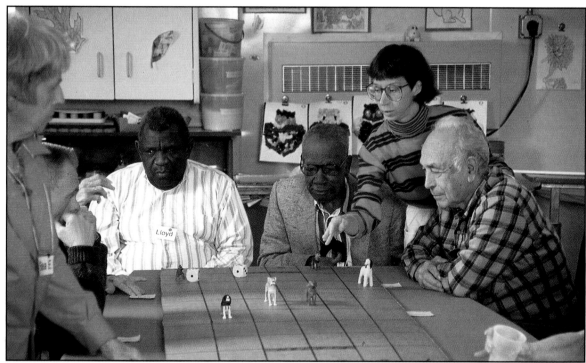

An adult day health care center can provide specific treatment needs for your residents, such as physical or occupational therapy, as well as the psychological benefits of meeting others with similar needs.

The purpose of home health agencies is to allow people to stay at home and receive basic homemaking services as well as skilled nursing care when needed. Hospice programs provide similar health services along with social services to those in the final stages of a terminal illness. The federal government funds hospice programs and home health care in some circumstances, but this care can be excessively expensive for private-pay individuals because of the administrative costs of the providing agencies. RCF residents can employ their own private duty nurses or aides for more intensive care. In all cases, evaluate residents with special health care needs to be sure that your license, if you have one, allows you to care for them.

Churches, Synagogues, and Other Religious Organizations

Churches, synagogues, and other religious organizations can be valuable resources for services, especially social services. One advantage of religious groups is that they are usually willing to visit

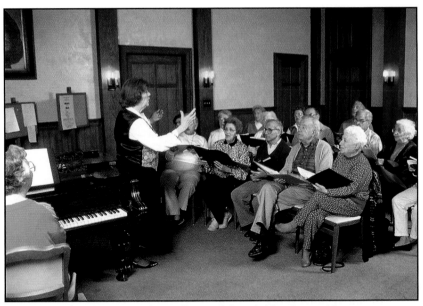

Religious organizations often offer social activities for residents.

your facility to provide religious services, music, or other meaningful activities for your residents. Religious participation on an individual basis, with visits from clergy or others, is a social service especially welcomed by some residents and should be available whenever possible.

Social and Civic Groups

Volunteer groups and service groups such as Hadassah, Lions Club, or Rotary can assist in providing activities for residents. Sometimes the best way to find vounteers is simply to "ask around." Those unable to provide help may know someone who can.

Associations

A resident with a specific disease or disability may require a level of understanding and care not readily available to the RCF, and it may be unrealistic to expect a resident's doctor to provide all the information needed (although that is a good place to start). The difference between a resident being able to stay in your facility and having to transfer to a nursing facility may rest on the specialized information available from national or local private agencies who focus on one particular disease or disability. There are associations for people with Alzheimer's disease, cancer, arthritis, amyotrophic lateral sclerosis (Lou Gehrig's disease), schizophrenia, mental retardation, and others. Appendix 1 lists some of these agencies.

Other Resources

Family members or friends may be willing to assist with personal care or taking the resident on an outing. When persons not in your employ are providing direct care services, you may be responsible for their actions. Check with legal counsel regarding potential liabilities. Even well-intentioned family members may lack the skill or patience required for the kind of assistance they are offering.

The best way to locate outside resources may be through a local elder services agency, often run by the city or county government. Although there is no single registry of agencies at this level, these agencies are listed in the phone book. State departments of aging, under a variety of titles, can offer assistance in locating local services. Appendix 1 lists sources for written materials and referrals. In some cases, information intended for those providing care to elderly persons at home can be useful.

Although it may be necessary to obtain outside assistance to meet important needs of your residents, it is equally important to organize your facility for optimal "in-home" care. Also, do not allow yourself to become dependent on people or agencies to help with ADLs and other health care needs at the expense of social services and activities. Most involved in the care of elderly residents living in even the most pleasant institutional environment consider social services and activities to be by far the most important services you can offer.

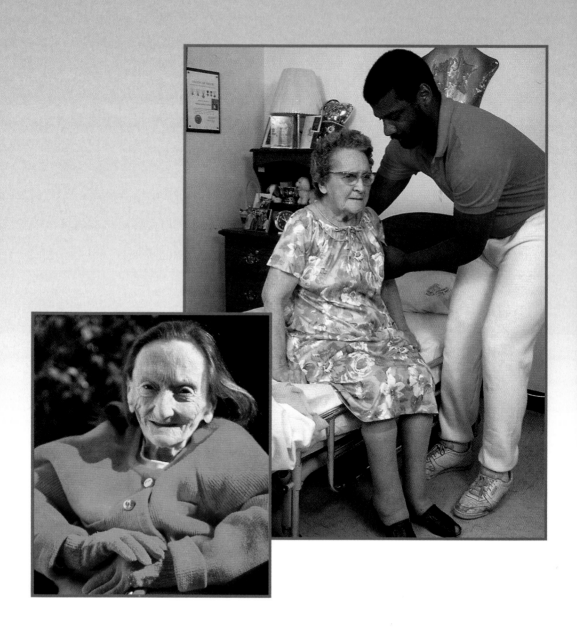

2

How to Plan Care

UNDERSTANDING YOUR RESIDENTS' NEEDS

Caring for the needs of elderly persons can be very fulfilling. Caregivers and managers who see improvement in resident health and well-being day by day receive more than just a salary for their efforts. Sometimes it is the residents most in need who give us the most satisfaction when they regain lost function or we see improvements in mental and emotional status. Unfortunately, caregivers also know the feeling of failure and frustration that comes from not being able to meet the needs of a particularly difficult-to-care-for resident; indeed, this frustration is also shared by nursing facility staff.

In assisted living environments, this often results when a resident who has lived a long time in a facility simply does not want to leave, even temporarily, for a higher level of care. This is usually due to the resident's satisfaction with his or her current living situation. In an elderly person it is also sometimes related to the not-unrealistic fear that he or she may never return to that previous level of care and facility. Staff members often develop the same sort of close attachments to residents, and they, too, are reluctant to take action when the resident needs a higher level of health care. This section will offer advice primarily on how to be sure you admit only those individuals for whom you can provide adequate care

Each of these women requires a different level of assistance. Assess your residents' needs carefully to be certain you can meet them.

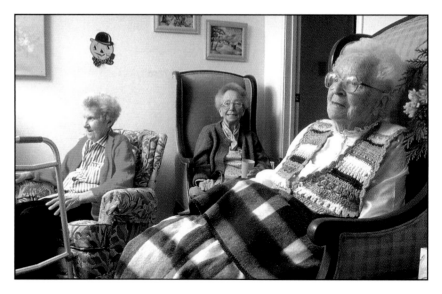

and on how to prepare yourself and your staff to meet those needs. Also included is information on what to do when your capabilities are exceeded.

THE INITIAL EVALUATION

The most important decision you will make about a resident is whether or not to accept that person into your care. If you use poor judgment, you may end up with someone whose needs you cannot meet. Besides potential legal liabilities, the wrong decision can create personal difficulties for the resident, his or her family, your staff, and you.

To be sure you have a clear idea of the kind of resident for whom you are able to care (what physical, social, dietary, and emotional services your facility can reasonably provide as well as any limits you have concerning language or culture) make an independent assessment of potential residents. Remember that the people who are trying to place potential residents may not always know the person's needs well and certainly will not know your capabilities as well as you do. Remember too that potential residents may present a biased picture of themselves, and an urgent need for placement may sometimes cause families and agencies to be less than forthcoming about the person they are trying to place.

It is important that you accept only residents for whom you can provide adequate services. Although the adequacy of services will need to include many things, direct care services are an especially important consideration. One way to be sure that you will be able to meet a prospective resident's needs is to complete a health status checklist for each applicant and compare the results with your capabilities. In some cases you will need the assistance of family members, the applicant's doctor, a transferring facility, or others. (*Caution:* Occasionally, families and transferring facilities are overly optimistic about the abilities of the person seeking admission to your facility.) Figure 2–1 offers a sample health status checklist to assist in your initial evaluation.

ADMISSION RECORD

Besides information concerning payment and next of kin, there are other items of information that will greatly assist you in meeting the resident's health and social needs that should be obtained as part of the resident's admission record.

Assuming that you have carefully screened a resident prior to admission, you should have a good idea of what his or her needs are going to be and of the services that you will need to provide. Document everything that you have learned and make sure that everyone caring for the resident agrees to the resident's plan of care.

The admission process is also the time to identify those who will be helping you to meet your new resident's needs. In many cases, people who are relatively independent want to assume responsibility for contacting others for what they need, but if you are taking care of older residents, there is always a chance that even the fairly independent individual will need more assistance later on. So it is a good idea to list the names, phone numbers, and addresses of the following:

- Interested relatives

- Friends

- Church, temple, or other religious group affiliations

- Volunteers

- Organizations resident may have belonged to that would offer support

- Health and welfare agency caseworker, if applicable

- Primary care doctor as well as all other doctors whom resident may be seeing; may simply be a central number for a clinic or health maintenance organization

- Dentist, chiropractor, or other health practitioner

- Pharmacy

STEPS TOWARD PROPER PLACEMENT

- Interview potential resident.

- Interview family and others, including doctors and other current or former caregivers who may understand the person's needs.

- Make sure the potential resident and those attempting to place him or her understand your facility's philosophy, capabilities, and limits.

Figure 2-1 **Health Status Checklist**

Yes   No

☐   ☐   **Does resident require assistance with bathing? If so, to what degree?**

    ☐ Partial only (please describe usual routine)

    ☐ Complete (please describe usual routine)

☐   ☐   **Is resident ever incontinent of urine? If so, how often?**

    ☐ Always or nearly always (measures taken)

    ☐ Occasionally (measures taken)

    ☐ Rarely (measures taken)

☐   ☐   **Is resident ever incontinent of stool? If so, how often?**
(*Note:* Such a resident can present difficult care problems.)

    ☐ Frequently or always (measures taken)

    ☐ Occasionally or rarely (measures taken)

☐   ☐   **Does resident need assistance with dressing? If so, to what degree?**

    ☐ Complete (usual routine)

    ☐ Partial only (usual routine)

☐   ☐   **What degree of assistance is required for mobility (ambulation)?**

    ☐ None

    ☐ Some

Complete list of all assistance needed (wheelchair, walker, cane, transfer only, stairs or not, etc.)

_____

_____

☐   ☐   **Does resident need assistance in eating? If so, describe:**

_____

_____

☐   ☐   **Does resident have speech difficulty or impairment? If so, describe:**

_____

_____

☐   ☐   **Does resident have hearing limitation? If yes, describe:**

_____

_____

Yes No

☐ ☐ **Check if resident uses a hearing aid and describe type, brand, and method of care.**

_____

_____

☐ ☐ **Does resident have non-correctable sight impairment? If so, describe:**

_____

_____

☐ ☐ **Does resident wear glasses?**

☐ ☐ **Does resident wear contact lenses? (If so, list type, care, and precautions.)**

_____

☐ ☐ **Does resident need assistance in caring for contact lenses?**

☐ ☐ **Does resident have an artificial limb, eye, or other prosthetic device/appliance? (If so, please describe type, care, and precautions.)**

_____

_____

☐ ☐ **Does resident need assistance in caring for the prosthesis/appliance?**

☐ ☐ **Does resident need assistance with medications? If yes, list names and doses and check needs.**

_____

_____

☐ Needs only reminder to take as ordered

☐ Needs medications prepared for self-administration

☐ Needs medications prepared for administration and some help in self-administering them

☐ ☐ **Does resident require special diet? If so, specify:**

_____

_____

☐ ☐ **Does resident suffer from a dementia or other mental disability that may affect the care and services provided? (If so, list type of disorder and specific needs.)**

_____

_____

☐ ☐ **Are there any other special needs that will require attention and services? If so, list:**

_____

_____

CARE PLANS

A resident's care plan can be used to list medical and related information, as well as specific steps and instructions to others that will be needed to assist your residents. For independent residents, the care plan may contain only the most basic information. For others, you may need to include a much more detailed list of problems and needs as well as the steps you and other caregivers will take to meet your obligations to those residents. Examples are illustrated in Figures 2–2 and 2–3.

Steps in Creating the Care Plan

• For each identified need, how will you provide the assistance needed? For example, how and when will you provide assistance in bathing? In visiting his or her doctor? In obtaining medications? The easiest way to handle this is to use a format where the disability, problem, or need is written down, and next to it the approaches you have decided to take.

• Do not try to do it all yourself. The resident and family or friends can help you identify what needs to be done, and how it should be accomplished. You will end up with a much better plan if others are involved in the process.

• Be as detailed as you need to be. For example, there may be a very specific procedure that caregivers need to go through to assist a resident to bathe. If you are going to provide substantial help with medications, it is very important that there be very specific directions on what the resident is to take, when, and perhaps even what foods can or cannot be eaten at the same time. Figure 2-4 Assessment of Medication Self-Adminstration Ability provides more information.

The care plan should be in writing, in a standard easy-to-follow format, and available to all staff involved in providing services to the resident.

To begin, you will need as much information about your resident as you can obtain. His or her likes, dislikes, physical and emotional needs, family or other social support, those involved in the provision of health care, including doctors, chiropractors, dentists, podiatrists, pharmacies, occupational, physical, and speech therapists, and any limitations on services related to financial status are all valuable in creating a plan of care for your resident. This information is usually kept in a separate file for each resident. You should keep separate all confidential information, such as specific financial data and any mental health information not actually needed for developing the care plan.

To encourage the standardization that will simplify staff training and improve efficiency and effectiveness in providing care, it will be useful to create a standard form—part to be completed by staff, other portions to be completed by the resident's family. Still other portions will need to be completed by providers such as doctors. See Sample Physician Communication Form in Figure 2–5.

Case Example

As an example, let us create a plan of care for Alice Carson, a newly admitted resident.

Alice is 82 years old. Until now, she lived at home in the same city as your facility. Three years ago her husband of 54 years died of a heart attack, and she has lived alone since then. She has a son and daughter-in-law, who have helped her take care of the house and financial matters, but her son recently took a job in a city about 100 miles away. Two daughters live in other states, and although one calls and writes regularly, she cannot afford to visit very often. A second son died in an automobile accident over 20 years ago.

Alice has lost some mobility and has some slurring of speech due to a "small stroke" 1 1/2 years ago, but she can be understood if one listens carefully. She had cataract surgery recently in her left eye.

Alice likes to shop, but does not like crowds. She is a dedicated reader, and likes to watch some television, but mostly just the late news. She has long had a habit of staying up late, getting up at 7 or 8 A.M.., and napping during the day. Sitting in the sun to read is another favorite pastime. Although she has outlived most of her friends, she still has occasional contact with some younger members of the local weavers guild, in which she used to be active until arthritis and her stroke prevented her from participating in weaving activities. She used to be active in a nearby Presbyterian church, but has not attended regularly for two or three years. For three years prior to her marriage, Alice was an elementary school teacher. She never went back to work after her four children were grown.

Alice has some right-side weakness and must use a cane or a walker to get about. She no longer drives, so is dependent on others for transportation. She must visit one doctor or another two or three times a month for her medical conditions, which include high blood pressure (currently well controlled), arthritis, glaucoma, a heart condition that involves an irregular heartbeat (arrhythmia) and some occasional chest pain, and diabetes, which is well controlled with diet and a medication she takes by mouth. In the last year, she has begun to develop parkinsonism, with some tremors and slight problems in mobility. Alice is a non-smoker, with no allergies, except to egg products. She is continent of bowel and bladder, although she must urinate frequently and has occasional minor bladder "leaks" on exertion or when she sneezes or laughs hard. In addition to eyeglasses, she wears hearing aids in both ears, although the results are mixed, and her left ear is the better of the two, with or without the hearing aid.

Alice is still "sharp" mentally, although she is sometimes confused, probably due in part to her hearing difficulty, and is forgetful enough that her son and daughter-in-law recently purchased a "medication reminder" device to help her remember to take her medications on time, something that has been a problem for her. Alice takes a variety of medications, including pilocarpine, timolol (Timoptic), and artificial tears for her eyes; furosemide, digoxin, diltiazem (Cardizem CD), nitroglycerin, and warfarin (Coumadin) for her heart condition; fluoxetine (Prozac) for depression; naproxen (Naprosyn) for arthritis; carbidopa/levodopa (Sinemet) for her parkinsonism; and glipizide (Glucotrol) for her diabetes. Alice sees a general practitioner, a rheumatologist for her arthritis, an ophthalmologist, and a cardiologist (heart specialist).

With the information available, and Alice's participation in the process, a good beginning plan of care can be created (Figure 2-2).

KEEPING RECORDS CURRENT

As with all of us, the needs of elderly people change over time. Often changes will occur much more quickly in the elderly, either due to an event such as a stroke or fall or just because the person is older. Mental, social, emotional, and physical status can all change rapidly. The caregiver has to be prepared to deal with sudden changes that warrant prompt attention, and to respond to more subtle changes requiring careful observation and thought.

The more detailed your initial data and plans are for an individual resident, the easier it will be for you to identify the kind of changes a resident may experience and when it is necessary to notify the resident's family or doctor. Any change may result in a need to make changes in your care plan and the methods you use to meet your residents' needs.

Obvious and sudden changes should be dealt with quickly, perhaps at first by a call to the resident's doctor. Doctors, dentists, and other health care professionals may identify additional changes for you after they have seen your resident.

Figure 2-2 **Sample Care Plan**

Shady Acres Manor
Resident Plan of Care

RESIDENT NAME: Alice Barbara Carson   **DOB**: 8/21/12   ☐ M ☒ F
RESPONSIBLE PARTY AND ADDRESS: Self
IN CASE OF EMERGENCY, NOTIFY: Alan Carson (Wife is Marie) **RELATIONSHIP:** Son
PHONE #: 399–4456   **ADDRESS:** 11245 East Hanover St.,Wilsonville (99945)
ALLERGIES: FOOD: Eggs   MEDICATIONS: None   OTHER: None

ADL: Dresses herself, but occasionally needs assistance with some clothing. Independent for toileting, eating, and bathing. Likes to stay up late and watch late news. Gets up around 7 to 8 A.M., likes to nap for about 45 minutes in the early afternoon. Ambulates independently, but uses cane & sometimes "tennis ball" walker. Is somewhat shaky, but knows to use railings and grab bars. Has used sleeping pills only rarely in the past. Eats all meals, but is a relatively light eater.

Plan:

(1) Resident will let staff know when she is expecting or is having difficulty with a particular item of clothing.

(2) She will remain independent for all other ADLs, with staff observing for further deterioration in mobility.

(3) Offer late A.M. breakfast and late evening snack if OK with her doctor.

SOCIAL SERVICES and ACTIVITIES: Resident is disappointed about her son and daughter-in-law moving and having to leave her home. She has not stayed in close touch with her friends in the last 2 or 3 years, especially since her stroke. She was a weaver for many years and has a fine collection of clothing and other articles she has woven over the years. She reads her Bible regularly, and asks about church activities. She is aware of her slight speech problem resulting from a stroke (she slurs some words and tends to talk softly), is sometimes irritated (possibly with herself) when people can't understand her, and feels badly when she can't hear others because of her hearing problem, especially in her right ear (she has hearing aids in both ears). Her occasional urinary incontinence "leaks" don't seem to bother her much ("It's a small price to pay for a good laugh!"). She needs glasses for reading and mobility. Likes hymns and "new age music," hates "acid rock."

Plan:

(1) Prefers to be called Alice or Mrs. Carson by persons of all ages.

(2) Contact her old weaver's guild to see if she can attend meetings without actually doing any weaving, and invite her friends from the guild to visit her. Ask Alice if we can put some of her weaving on display and ask if she would be interested in leading a discussion on weaving for other interested residents. Introduce Alice to Mrs. Andrews and Mrs. O'Hara, both of whom are interested in weaving.

(3) Contact minister at the Briarwood Presbyterian Church about services that she could attend and see if there is a possibility of someone from the church visiting.

(4) Encourage son and wife to visit whenever possible and take Alice on an excursion.

Continued on the following page

Continued from the previous page

(5) Encourage Alice to take advantage of the Elder Shopping bus.

(6) Listen patiently when she is talking; don't show impatience or try to finish sentences for her. Re-state what she says if there is any doubt. Speak clearly, but don't shout. Speak toward her left ear if you are having a problem, and let Alice see your lips when speaking. If she is incontinent, don't show alarm; use good humor to help her to change.

(7) Remind Alice of facility library and library van visit every Wed.

(8) Check walker occasionally to be sure it is working correctly.

(9) Resident has TV and CD player in room, both with separate earphones.

DIET:

(1) Diabetic; standard diabetic diet as ordered by Dr.

(2) "No Egg Products" warning on her diet card.

(3) Offer late night snack as per diet menu and put on late breakfast schedule.

(4) Likes: meats, fish, and poultry; low carbohydrate desserts, nuts, most vegetables and starches, an occasional beer or glass of wine.

(5) Dislikes: lima beans, eggplant, cabbage.

MEDICAL:

Alice is on Coumadin, a blood thinner that needs to be carefully monitored with frequent blood tests. Any new medication, or stopping any current medication, will mean that she will need extra blood tests to prevent serious bleeding or inadequate thinning of her blood. Her primary care doctor needs to be informed of any change in medication, including the use of over-the-counter medications. Any new bruising or signs of bleeding require contacting the doctor, as they may reflect her blood being too thin. Certain foods that contain vitamin K may also interfere with this medication, and the doctor should be asked if there are any special dietary concerns.

Doctors—Phone number and address:

1. Harry Green, MD 887–5569; 127 Oak St. (general practice)

2. Sandra Arnold, MD (920) 458–3394; 3200 Park Plaza, Ste. 33, Littletown (eye doctor)

3. J.J. Rhajanivani, MD 887–2299; 155 Oak St. (cardiologist)

4. Podiatrist: Alfred Hanover, DPM (920) 443–3330; 1985 Harrington Dr. (visits Shady Acres monthly)

Pharmacy—Specialized Care Pharmacy 887–2222; 199 Oak St. (delivery 7 days a week). She will call for refills.

Hearing Aid—Hansen's Auditory Center 887–3006

Plan:

Resident goes to Dr. Green at Doctor's Medical Center every month for check-up and blood tests. Prefers Tuesdays; next appointment made on each visit. Dr. is very cooperative regarding completion of doctor visit form.

Wants only reminders now for medications (schedule attached) but admits to past problems in not taking meds correctly.

Date of entry: _____

Figure 2-3 **Sample Care Plan**

Shady Acres Manor
Resident Plan of Care

RESIDENT NAME: Stephen De La Torre   **DOB:**   5/18/18   M [X] F [ ]

RESPONSIBLE PARTY AND ADDRESS: George De La Torre
124A Gordon Way
Betterstown, 99929

IN CASE OF EMERGENCY, NOTIFY: George De La Torre (above)

RELATIONSHIP: Son
ADDRESS: 124A Gordon Way, Betterstown 99929
PHONE #: (222) 518–0046

ALLERGIES: FOOD: None   MEDICATIONS: None   OTHER: None

ADL: Physically independent, but forgets to bathe and brush teeth sometimes; gets clothes mixed up.

Plan:

(1) West wing aides to set up bathing schedule and remind him to bathe.

(2) Remind him of dental care needs during morning and evening medication visits.

(3) Check on morning visit to be sure clothing appropriate.

(4) Housekeeping will tidy up clothing as needed.

SOCIAL SERVICES and ACTIVITIES: Played pro football for a year or 2, then worked for a beer distributor for many years. Likes watching TV, especially football and basketball and talk shows. Likes to go walking with others, but he is in very good shape and most residents cannot keep up with him. Non-smoker last 40+ years. Widowed 15 years ago after 25-year marriage; keeps wife's picture in room, but has apparently adjusted well. Doesn't like female residents "nagging" him about his appearance or loud TV (he has some hearing loss and hearing aid in left ear, which he wears off and on). Likes to talk about football. Catholic, likes to go to mass on Sundays, but no other participation. Expects to be called Mr. De La Torre, but asks staff he knows well to call him Steve. Is forgetful, but retains reasonable short-term memory. Doesn't care much for excursions unless they involve walking.

Plan:

(1) Consider room assignment with Mr. GS, who likes sports on TV.

(2) Introduce him to Mrs. FW, whose husband was a college football coach.

(3) Remind him to wear his hearing aid when watching TV in the living room.

(4) Check Mall Walkers club to see if someone can pick him up.

(5) Encourage him to go with staff noontime walkers.

(6) Church bus to St. Anthony's.

Continued on the following page

Continued from the previous page

DIET:

(1) Eats everything, but likes simple foods best.

(2) Drinks lots of coffee.

(3) Likes beer in the evening (family keeps him supplied).

MEDICAL:

Gordon's Hearing Center for hearing aid problems.

Dr. Guy Allen is eye doctor for glaucoma (Downtown Eye Clinic, 521–1020).

Dr. Marti Barbera family medicine, Doctors Medical Clinic on Virginia Street; 521–1122 (see MD communication form).

Dentist is Ernesto Rivera on 14th and Gary Avenue (428–2540).

Plan:

(1) No restrictions on activities.

(2) Needs to be reminded to take meds (see schedule). Only takes blood pressure pills in A.M., takes eye drops morning and night.

Date of entry: _____

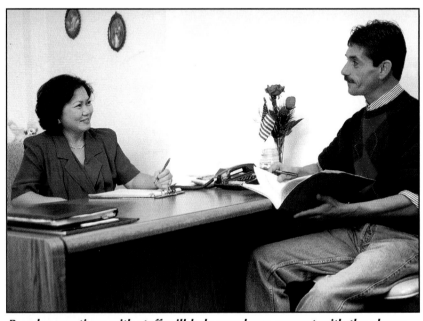

Regular meetings with staff will help you keep current with the changing needs of your residents.

Figure 2-4 **Assessment of Medication Self-Administration Ability**

Resident:_____ **Rm #:**_____ **Date:**_____

Person(s) Involved in Assessment (Include resident and family members if applicable):

_____

_____

List All Medications Used:

_____

_____

ASSESSMENT:

1. Cognitive Ability:

  ☐ Adequate for complete self-administration

  ☐ Limited: Needs reminders or may take extra doses

  ☐ Not competent to manage own medications

2. Physical Limitations (e.g., arthritis, lack of mobility):

_____

_____

3. Other Limitations Based on Nature of Drug or Resident Condition:

_____

_____

4. List Any Special Need for Complete Self-Administration of One or More Medications:

_____

_____

Ordering Prescriptions From Pharmacy:

  ☐ Assistance needed

  ☐ No assistance

Administration of Medications:

  ☐ Resident to store and manage all of own medications.

  ☐ As above with reminders for all routine doses, careful check of quantities on reorder.

  ☐ Resident to store and manage only (list drugs) _____
    All others centrally stored and assistance provided.

  ☐ All medications centrally stored and assistance provided for all doses.

  ☐ Other (explain) _____

Figure 2-5 **Sample Physician Communication Form**

Sunnyside Assisted Living Care Center
"Where Caring is a Way of Life"
121 Gary Ln Carterville (111) 773–3329

RESIDENT NAME:_____DATE:_____

DOCTOR'S NAME & PHONE #:_____

CURRENT COMPLAINTS/PROBLEMS:

_____

_____

_____

CURRENT MEDICATIONS:

☐ See attached dose schedule

☐ Other:

_____

_____

_____

DOCTOR'S INSTRUCTIONS

(Please attach any prescriptions and let us know what care we should provide):

_____

_____

_____

Signature:_____Date:_____

Less obvious changes may not be easily seen by busy caregivers, but may be identified through a routine, comprehensive review process. Set aside some time each month to review a number of your residents, and encourage all your staff to provide input. In larger facilities, stagger the reviews so that only a few residents at a time are reviewed. The reviews can be brief and held in conjunction with some other activity or meeting involving the staff.

Compare everyone's impressions against the information you have in the resident's file to see if you need to make changes. For some residents, this review may be performed annually; for others, a quarterly review may be needed. Plan a review for new residents shortly after your first plan of care has been developed so that you can modify the plan based on what you now know about the resident. If, as a result of these reviews, you determine that there have been significant changes in the resident, be sure to inform others, including the resident's doctor and family.

Remember always to involve the resident and, if possible, the family when you think a change in services is warranted. It may take some negotiation between you and the resident or between the resident and family for the resident to agree with your recommendations.

Even health professionals often dread the prospect of writing "progress notes" or assessments of residents. Many of us try to avoid writing anything at all! Especially for caregivers with limited formal education, the trick is to write down just what you would have said aloud about the resident. Do not worry about grammar or spelling; just get the information down on paper. If your handwriting is especially bad, print. Remember that doctors are among the highest educated health care providers, and most of them cannot read what they write!

Finally, be careful not to include derogatory statements that you would regret if the record were read by the resident or family or if it ever went to court.

WHEN A RESIDENT NEEDS MORE CARE THAN YOU CAN PROVIDE

One of the hardest things for both RCF operators and their residents is to have to admit that the facility can no longer meet all of the resident's needs. In some cases this decision is "hurried along" by state or county limits on the kind of care a facility can provide.

Often, residents must go to a higher level of care in a hospital or nursing facility because of a sudden or serious change in mental

Figure 2-6 **Interfacility Transfer Form**

Name_____ Gender_____ DOB_____

Transferring facility_____ Religion_____

Address_____ Phone_____

Dates of stay_____

SS#_____ Medicare#_____ Insurance#_____

Responsible relative/guardian_____

Address_____ Phone_____

Physician_____ Phone_____ Nurse_____ Phone_____

Other physician_____

Date/time of transfer_____ Recent vital signs_____

Reason for transfer_____

Physician orders on transfer_____

Hospital/facilities discharged within 60 days_____

Advance directives_____

Critical care plan_____

Allergies_____ Immunizations_____

Medications_____

Other treatments (PT, resp, diet, etc.)_____

Past medical history_____

Primary diagnosis_____

Secondary diagnosis_____

Surgical history_____

Tabacco/alcohol_____

BASELINE INFORMATION

	Ambulation_____	
Activities of Daily Living	Bathing_____	Transfer_____
	Dressing_____	Continence_____
	Toileting_____	Feeding_____
Disabilities	Amputation_____	Contracture_____
	Paralysis_____	Decubitus ulcer_____
Impairments	Speech_____	Vision_____
	Hearing_____	Sensation_____
Usual Mental Status	Alert_____	Oriented_____
	Wanders_____	Combative_____
	Confused_____	Withdrawn_____
	Other_____	

Appliances/supports (e.g., wheelchair, cane, walker, prosthesis)_____

Other information to emergency providers_____

Reprinted with permission from Sanders, Arthur B. (1996)., *Emergency Care of the Elder Person.* St. Louis, MO: Beverly Cracom Publications

status, a stroke, a fall resulting in a fracture, or a serious infection. In most of these cases, unless progressive deterioration is anticipated, the goal is to return the resident to the RCF level of care.

Problems and uncertainty occur more often when the change in the resident has taken place over a long period of time, and the resident is adamant about staying with you even though you know that you can no longer provide the care and services he or she needs. Depending on resources available and any licensing restrictions, it may be possible to provide certain kinds of special care through home health or visiting nurse agencies. If that is not possible, RCF caregivers can help their residents adjust to the inevitable change to a nursing facility or another higher level of care.

Just as you need good, comprehensive information on residents when they first come to you, so will the nursing facility, hospital, etc., which will now be providing care to the resident. Even if you are not asked for the information, give the new facility any information concerning the resident that you think will be useful (Figure 2-6). Of particular value will be information on mental, emotional, and social status and needs. Always ask for the same kind of feedback from hospitals or nursing facilities and doctors when residents come back to you.

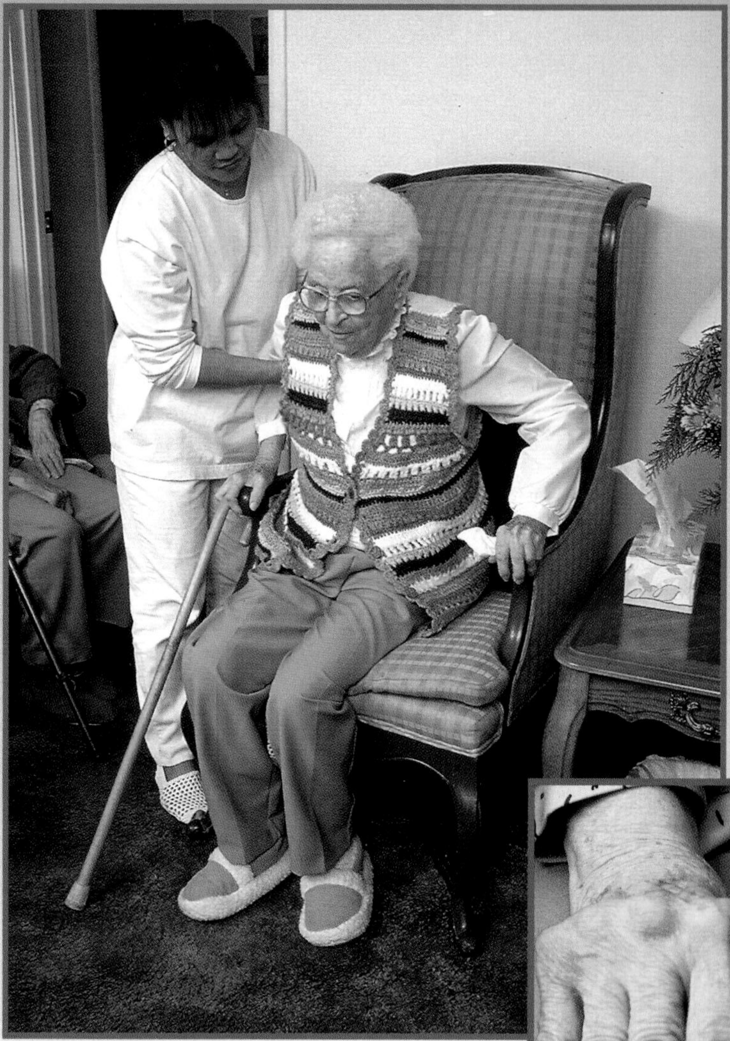
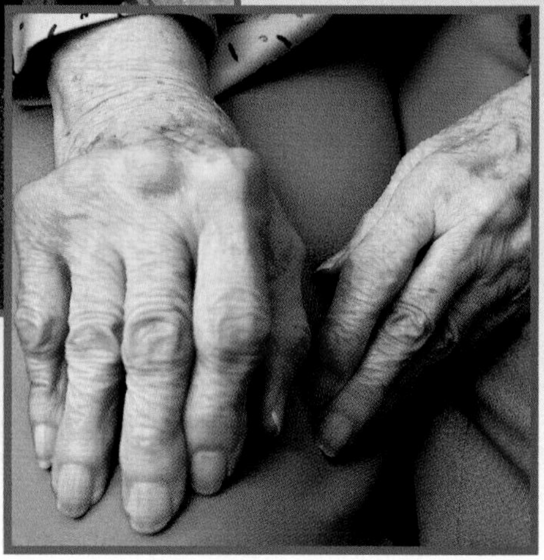

SECTION

3

Common Health Problems

When illness occurs in a family, the level of understanding and support from family members can significantly affect the success of medical treatment by ensuring that appropriate medical attention is obtained, that the treatment plan is followed, and that any problems or changes in the individual's condition are reported. The same is true in the residential care facility (RCF), where caregivers may encounter a variety of acute and chronic illnesses among their residents.

No one expects you to diagnose illness or to prescribe and administer treatment (remember, you are not legally qualified or permitted to do so). But you can help your residents achieve the greatest possible benefit from prescribed treatment plans and help ensure their safety and well-being by recognizing the need for medical attention. Specific responsibilities may include simply helping a resident remember to take prescribed medications, but you also may be faced with circumstances that require immediate medical attention.

This section will help prepare you for these responsibilities by identifying common health problems among elderly people, explaining bodily processes and organ functions that are affected, and outlining steps you can take to promote your residents' health and safety and to ensure effective treatment when medical intervention is required.

Generic drugs presented in the medication checklists are lowercase. Brand name drugs are capitalized.

ABDOMINAL PAIN

The abdomen is the part of the body often referred to by lay-persons as "the stomach" or "the belly." The term abdomen actually refers to the area of the body below the breastbone and above the pubic area. It contains the digestive organs—the stomach, intestines, liver, and gallbladder, as well as the spleen and kidneys. Given all these organs and its relatively large size, many different problems can cause abdominal pain. This pain can be severe and sudden or it can be a long-term problem. It can be sharp and knife-like, dull or crampy. It can be a sign of serious trouble or just another ache or pain that one must learn to live with. The characteristics of the pain help to determine whether or not it is an emergency, and help the doctor determine the cause of the pain.

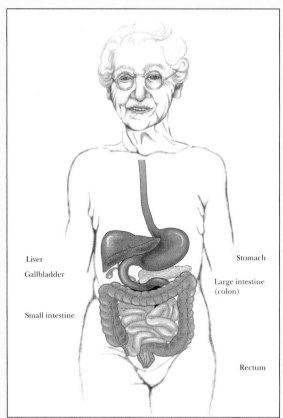

Abdominal organs

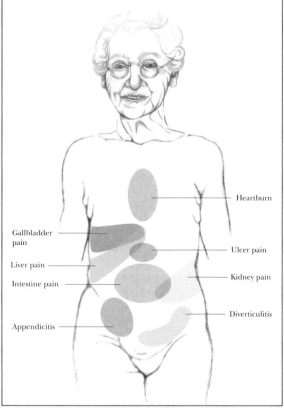

Locations and potential significance of pain

What It Is   Pain is often a warning from the body that "something's wrong." Pain is a way that the brain interprets signals carried by nerves from elsewhere in the body. Nerves that are stretched, damaged, or inflamed send a signal that the brain interprets as pain. The organs in the abdomen are richly supplied with nerves, and many, many processes can stimulate these nerves into sending the message of pain.

Abdominal pain generally means some structure in the abdomen is being disturbed—it could be an inflamed stomach or appendix, or a tear in the huge blood vessel that passes through the abdomen (called the aorta). It could be a gallstone passing through a narrow tube connecting the gallbladder to the bowel. It could be painful cramps of the bowel, or an ulcer in the stomach. It could be something as relatively simple as a spicy food irritating the lining of the stomach or hard, dry stool distending the walls of the bowel. It is the doctor's challenge to figure it out.

Types and Locations of Abdominal Pain

Types	Locations
• Sharp (knife-like, stabbing) • Dull • Burning • Crampy • Gnawing	• Generalized • Right upper abdomen— often related to gallbladder • Right lower abdomen—may be appendix • Left lower abdomen—may be due to constipation or rectal disease • Below naval—may be bladder distention

Health Impact   The importance of abdominal pain relates to whatever is causing it. The pain may be an important warning of a catastrophe about to happen inside the belly, or it may be a long-standing problem that requires long-term management. A useful way to evaluate abdominal pain is to think of it as acute or sudden pain and ongoing chronic pain.

VARIATIONS

Associated Signs and Symptoms
- Nausea or vomiting
- Diarrhea or bright red blood in the stool
- Black, tarry, sticky stool
- A pale, "pasty" appearance of the skin, often noticed first in the face

Dangerous Changes in Symptoms
- New onset of abdominal pain, especially if it is severe
- Pain that becomes constant or increases dramatically in severity
- Pain associated with vomiting, fever, or bloody bowel movements
- Pain associated with feeling faint or light-headed

Sudden vs Chronic Abdominal Pain

Sudden	Chronic
Passing a gallstone	Inflamed stomach or bowel
Perforated ulcer in stomach or small bowel	Chronic or recurrent ulcers in the stomach or small bowel
Ruptured aorta	Cancer of the stomach, gallbladder, bowel, or kidney
Obstruction of the passage of urine with sudden distention of the urinary bladder	Constipation
Inflammation of the liver (hepatitis)	Bacterial or viral infection of the bowel
Infection or inflammation of appendix (appendicitis)	Radiation damage from radiation therapy
Infection of the gallbladder (cholecystitis)	

ALERT

Abrupt, severe, generalized abdominal pain needs to be reported to the doctor as soon as possible. Do not try to treat severe abdominal pain yourself with home remedies, antacids, laxatives, or by using another resident's medication.

MEDICATION CHECKLIST

The medical treatment of abdominal pain is complicated by the fact that so many different processes cause abdominal pain. Needless to say, the proper treatment depends on what you are treating. Many of the acute or sudden causes of abdominal pain are treated with surgery rather than with medicines.

Antacids. Antacids neutralize stomach acid, often improving the pain related to ulcers or stomach inflammation. Common examples include mixtures of magnesium and aluminum hydroxide (Maalox, Mylanta, Riopan), calcium carbonate (Tums, Titrolac), and aluminum hydroxide (Amphogel).

Acid-Blocking Drugs. These medications actually block the stomach from making acid, and are used to improve pain related to ulcers, heartburn or stomach inflammation. Common examples include cimetidine (Tagamet), ranitidine (Zantac), famotidine (Pepcid), and omeprazole (Prilosec). Both Tagamet and Pepcid are now available without a prescription. Sucralfate (Carafate) does not block acid production, but by coating the stomach lining it also is used to heal ulcers.

Antispasmodics. These medications are used to decrease crampy bowel pain. They are generally not used until the causes of the pain are investigated and the very dangerous causes of abdominal pain have been excluded. Common examples include belladonna (hyoscyamine, atropine, and scopolamine) combined with the sedative drug phenobarbital (Donnatal and many others). These drugs can cause drowsiness, difficulty urinating, blurry vision, and confusion in elderly persons.

Laxatives. See section on constipation for a discussion of these drugs.

Narcotic Analgesics (Pain Medication). These strong and potentially addictive pain drugs are generally reserved for abdominal pain that cannot be relieved with less potent drugs. A commonly used drug is morphine (MS-Contin, Oramorph-SR, and others), but other narcotics such as Fentanyl (Duralgesic) and Hydromorphone (Dilaudid) are also used. All of these drugs have constipation and drowsiness as side-effects.

YOUR ROLE

For new abdominal pain or pain that changes in character or is associated with the dangerous symptoms identified earlier, contact the doctor immediately. For long-standing abdominal pain, observe the resident for any changes, and provide adequate, nutritious food to help prevent poor nutrition.

Medical Treatment

- Evaluation either in the emergency department, doctor's office, or by phone
- Hospitalization as needed
- Medications
- Surgery to repair or remove damaged organs
- Special diet

Residential Care Actions

- Evaluate any resident complaining of abdominal pain.
- If pain is new or pain has changed in character, contact doctor.
- Discuss resident's use of aspirin and other non-prescription pain medications with the doctor.
- Monitor use of antacids or other medications resident takes for pain.
- Encourage fluid intake and fiber for residents with constipation.
- Limit alcohol use.

 DIET TIPS

- Bland diet only if prescribed by physician.
- Extra fluid and fiber in diet if resident is constipated.
- Dietary supplements or small, frequent meals if appetite is poor.
- Alcohol use should be avoided.
- Many medications should not be given at the same time as antacids. If in doubt, ask the doctor!

FOR YOUR RECORDS

Health History

- History of ulcer disease or abdominal surgery
- Medication use including aspirin and other non-prescription drugs
- Alcohol use

Current Needs
- Weight monitoring
- Monitoring of medication use, including antacids
- Monitoring pattern when resident wakes up at night with pain, if pain occurs in relation to meals, or if particular foods or alcohol use trigger episodes of pain

COMMON QUESTIONS

When should I call the doctor?

The new development of abdominal pain should always be brought to the attention of the doctor. Any change in the nature of long-standing pain, or any of the dangerous symptoms listed earlier, should prompt quick attention from the doctor.

What is an ulcer?

An ulcer is a disruption to the protective inner lining of the stomach or small bowel. It can be painless or painful, and can cause serious problems like bleeding, or even a complete perforation of the stomach or bowel leading to digestive juices spilling into the body cavity, causing severe pain or death. Ulcers can be caused by drugs that damage the lining of the stomach, including aspirin and many common anti-inflammatory drugs used for arthritis. Another cause of ulcers is a bacterial infection of the lining of the gut. A less common but very serious cause of ulceration is an underlying cancer of the stomach.

Why did the doctor give antibiotics for the resident's ulcer?

Doctors now believe that many ulcers are related to an infection of the stomach. To best heal the ulcer, antibiotics may be used in addition to the antacids and medications listed.

Why does a resident with an abdominal problem not need to be on a bland diet?

Although bland diets were previously used for a variety of ailments affecting the stomach and bowels, they are now rarely needed. The doctor lets the patient decide if a particular food bothers the stomach. Appetizing food helps prevent malnutrition, and bland food is often unappetizing to the resident.

What are adhesions?

When surgery, infection, radiation, or injury causes damage to the delicate tissues lining the abdomen, tough scars can form that connect different parts of the lining of the abdomen to segments of the bowel. If a loop of bowel gets caught in a narrow area between some of these adhesions, the bowel's blood supply gets choked off and severe pain can result. This may require surgery to free the trapped loop of the bowel.

ANGINA AND CORONARY ARTERY DISEASE

Angina is the name given to a type of pain that occurs when the heart is not receiving enough blood to supply the heart's oxygen needs. Most often, the cause is a build up of fatty deposits in the blood vessel walls. The blood vessels that supply the heart are called *coronary arteries,* and the fatty deposits cause *coronary artery disease.*

Fatty deposits called plaque, can cause obstruction of an artery.

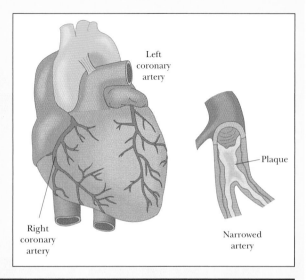

Left coronary artery

Plaque

Right coronary artery

Narrowed artery

What It Is

Fatty deposits in the blood vessels, called *atherosclerosis,* develop as a result of several factors. The most common factor is heredity in which a type of carrier protein causes more fat to be deposited in the blood vessels. The risk of having angina or a heart attack, therefore, is greater if this type of heart disease runs in your family. Other risk factors include certain medical conditions, particularly diabetes, and gender (while men develop this problem earlier in life than women, women are not spared from this disease, and risk increases after menopause). Factors that can be modified include diet, exercise, and smoking. By limiting the fat in our diet, keeping physically active, and not smoking, we can dramatically lower our chance of developing this problem.

Health Impact

Imagine that every time you tried to walk briskly or lift a heavy object you had a strong, crushing pain in your chest. This is what many persons with angina experience, although medications can help relieve the pain for most people. However, knowing that pain is likely to occur with certain activities can be a problem by itself, causing a person to limit exercise and even common activities like walking or bathing. Additionally, if the disease progresses, the heart may become so deprived of oxygen that a heart attack occurs.

The term *heart attack* means that part of the heart muscle dies.

VARIATIONS

One of the important characteristics of angina is not necessarily related to how severe the pain is, but rather to how frequent the pain is. Many residents with angina will have predictable pain when doing a particularly strenuous activity, but the character and severity of their pain is always about the same. This is called *stable angina*, and it usually is managed with medications. When angina changes over a few hours or days, either by becoming more severe, spreading to other parts of the body, or becoming more common or occurring with little or no physical activity, it is called *unstable angina*. Unstable angina should be considered an emergency and requires contacting the resident's doctor.

Another important variation to understand is that angina does not always cause chest pain. Sometimes the body's reaction to inadequate blood flow to the heart will cause nausea, dizziness, or shortness of breath. This is called *variant angina*. Such symptoms occur under the same circumstances as the more common form of angina, such as during physical or emotional stress.

Early Symptoms
- Mild chest pain or odd feelings in the chest when exercising, or when emotionally upset
- A feeling of chest pressure or tightness
- Shortness of breath
- Sweating
- A sense of impending doom or death
- Pain in the jaw or left arm

Advanced Symptoms
- Chest pain or pressure when doing only mild exercise
- Chest pain or pressure when at rest
- Reluctance to perform common activities due to fear of chest pain

Potential Problems and Complications
- Heart attack
- Sudden death

ALERT

Chest pain or pressure that is more severe or prolonged than usual or that does not respond to medication needs to be reported to the doctor immediately.

MEDICATION CHECKLIST

Nitrates. Nitrates increase blood flow to the heart. They can be used under the tongue (to work extra fast), as a skin patch, as a spray, and as pills. Common examples include nitroglycerin (which is available as tablets, a spray, and ointments) and isosorbide dinitrate (Isordil). It is very important that nitroglycerin tablets be stored in their original, dark and dry container. Nitroglycerin loses its effect after time, and new pills are needed even if that means throwing away unused pills.

Vasodilators. Vasodilators are drugs that expand the blood vessels, letting blood flow more easily, thereby easing the heart's work, decreasing chest pain, and lowering the risk of a heart attack. Examples are calcium channel blockers, beta blockers, and hydralazine. Common calcium channel blocking drugs are nifedipine (Adalat CC, Procardia XL), diltiazem (Cardizem), and verapamil (Calan, Isoptin). Common beta blockers are propranolol (Inderal), metoprolol (Lopressor, Toprol), and atenolol (Tenormin).

YOUR ROLE

Your role for a resident who is having severe angina or who has chest pain for the first time is to obtain professional help immediately. This usually means calling 911, but some residents who have other medical conditions such as dementia or cancer may not be best served by intensive hospital care. In such cases, the doctor will have had to instruct you in advance. If you have no instructions, you should call for help immediately. Sometimes the symptoms of a heart attack are subtle or confusing. If you have any doubt, contact the doctor for guidance.

After the initial medical treatment, a resident with angina is likely to take a variety of medications and supervision is important to monitor side-effects. The resident may need to keep nitroglycerin tablets or spray available at all times, so that medication can be given as quickly as possible when angina occurs. Physical activity may have to be limited, but in general it will be important to clarify with the doctor specific recommendations and restrictions. A special diet may be part of treatment, and it will be important for you to be sure your staff understands specific requirements and restrictions.

Medical Treatment
- Nitroglycerin tablets and other medications
- Limitations of physical activity
- Hospitalization
- Surgery to open blockages in blood vessels

 DIET TIPS

- A low-fat, low-sodium (salt) diet is often prescribed by the doctor. Animal fats are usually limited to specific amounts, and a particular fat, called cholesterol, may also be limited. If a special diet is prescribed, be sure your kitchen staff fully understands it. (For example, fatty or salty snacks like potato chips are usually limited.)
- Extra fiber and fluids may be recommended if constipation is present.
- Dietary supplements or small, frequent meals may be recommended if appetite is poor.
- Alcohol use should be discussed with the doctor. One or two drinks may be permitted, unless a particular medication cannot be used in combination with alcohol. If in doubt, ask!

FOR YOUR RECORDS

Health History
- Previous heart attack
- High blood pressure
- Medication use
- Alcohol use

Current Needs
- Weight monitoring
- Maintaining or regaining normal functional status
- Avoiding activities known to produce chest pain

COMMON QUESTIONS

How long can someone live with coronary artery disease?
Although coronary artery disease leads to heart attacks and can kill, when treated successfully people can live for many years with the disease. When angina cannot be treated successfully with medications, surgery can open blocked coronary arteries in many residents. It should be noted that many people who have severe narrowing of the blood vessels to the heart do not have any chest pain. The first sign of coronary artery disease can be sudden death from a heart attack. This results in a somewhat confusing situation in which one resident with severe angina may live many, many years, while another resident without angina may suddenly die from a heart attack!

Why does the chest pain sometimes occur when the resident is doing physical work?
The muscle walls of the heart need more oxygen during exercise than they do while resting. Often, blood vessels narrowed by fatty deposits allow enough blood flow to supply the needs of the heart muscle while resting, but cannot open enough to allow the needed increase for exercise. In this situation, angina pain occurs only during exercise.

What level of activity is appropriate for a resident with angina?
Even short periods of inactivity can lead to a permanent loss of strength and balance. In general, residents should stay as active as possible. Angina may be a limiting factor, however, and you should discuss activity recommendations with the doctor. Sometimes, a resident will be instructed to take a nitroglycerin tablet immediately before an activity, to prevent angina pain that might otherwise occur.

ANKLE SWELLING

Ankle swelling is an abnormal increase in the size of one or both ankles due to a buildup of excess fluid in the tissues.

What It Is

The heart's forceful pumping normally works against gravity to keep blood and other body fluids from "pooling" in the ankles and feet. When the heart is weakened, however, as in congestive heart failure, or when blood vessel disease affects the legs, gravity will pull more fluid into the lower extremities, and the circumference of the ankles may increase dramatically. This excess fluid is called *edema*. An indentation can sometimes be left when a fingertip is pressed against the skin. This is called pitting edema.

Health Impact

Swelling of the ankles can be uncomfortable and can lead to dry, cracked skin that is easily infected. Swollen legs can be heavy and can contribute to the risk of falling. The stretched skin over the ankles can be easily injured, and skin sores or open areas can develop. In severe cases, fluid can leak out of these open areas, and drain down the leg. Problems related to the water building up in other body tissues are discussed in the section on congestive heart failure.

VARIATIONS

Early Symptoms

- Ankle swelling that develops as the day goes on, but disappears overnight
- Enlarged purple leg veins
- Increased urination at night

Progressive Symptoms

- Swelling of the lower legs and feet that persists all day
- Dry, scaly, or cracked skin over ankles and lower legs
- Shortness of breath

Potential Problems and Complications

- Skin sores or ulcers
- Fluid "weeping" from breaks in the skin

ALERT

Worsening shortness of breath or increased swelling of legs needs to be reported to the doctor as soon as possible. Infection of the skin is another potentially serious problem associated with swollen ankles, and the doctor should be informed promptly if redness, increased warmth, or new tenderness of the leg develops.

MEDICATION CHECKLIST

Diuretics. Diuretics are commonly called "water pills," because they help get rid of excess salt *and* water. They can limit the swelling of the legs and the collection of water in the lungs. Common examples include furosemide (Lasix), hydrochlorothiazide, and triamterene/hydrochlorothiazise (Dyazide, Maxzide).

Digoxin. Digoxin is a plant extract that helps strengthen the heart and slow the heartbeat. Too much digoxin however can cause nausea or dangerously irregular heartbeats.

Vasodilators. Vasodilators expand the blood vessels, letting blood flow more easily and easing the heart's work. Examples are the ACE inhibitors and hydralazine (see section on angina).

Analgesics. Analgesics are also called pain medications and are used to help relieve pain related to a swollen, injured ankle. These medications are reviewed in the section on pain.

YOUR ROLE

Swollen ankles can be a minor inconvenience or a sign of a major medical problem. Your job is to contact the doctor if a resident develops swollen ankles. If only one ankle is swollen, and there is pain or a bruise, obtain medical attention as soon as possible to prevent further injury or a dangerous fall. If both ankles are swollen and no pain is present, inform the doctor at the next visit. Be sure to keep a record of the resident's weight to help the doctor treat this problem.

If the problem is the result of congestive heart failure, there is usually serious damage to the heart. Treatment is directed at improving heart function, and the swollen ankles improve as the heart pumps more effectively. Ankle swelling can also be a side effect of certain medications, including certain heart and blood pressure medications. In these cases, the doctor may decide to change a resident's medication.

Medical Treatment

- Elastic stockings to improve circulation
- Diuretics (also called water pills)
- Medication to help the heart pump more effectively
- Supplemental oxygen
- Surgery, in selected cases, to repair blood vessel problems

Residential Care Actions

- Sodium (salt) restricted diet
- Assistance with elastic stockings
- Elevating the legs
- Weight monitoring
- Prompt reporting of any new shortness of breath, skin infection, or other change in the resident's condition
- Frequent inspection of the skin of the resident's legs and feet
- Ensuring regular visits to the podiatrist (foot doctor)

 DIET TIPS

- Low-sodium (salt) diet as prescribed by doctor
- Extra potassium in diet *only if prescribed*
- Extra fiber and fluids if constipation is present
- Dietary supplements or small, frequent meals if appetite is poor

FOR YOUR RECORDS

Health History

- History of ankle swelling
- History of varicose veins or other circulation problems in the legs
- History of skin problems in the legs
- Medication use

Current Needs
- Weight monitoring
- Skin care
- Extra pillows for sleep
- Easy access to bathroom or commode because of urgent need to urinate at night
- Help putting on elastic stockings or leg dressings
- Steps to minimize urinary incontinence

COMMON QUESTIONS

How much should swollen legs be elevated?
If the doctor recommends elevating the legs, ideally the lowest part of the leg should be higher than the heart. This means that just putting the legs on a footstool while the resident sits is not high enough. You may need several pillows as well as a footstool to achieve proper elevation of the legs.

Why does the doctor not prescribe enough diuretics to completely eliminate ankle swelling?
Side effects from diuretics can make it dangerous to attempt to completely eliminate swelling.

What level of activity is appropriate for the resident with swollen ankles?
Even short periods of inactivity can lead to a permanent loss of strength and balance. Residents should stay as active as possible. If the swelling is related to poor circulation in the veins, walking may help pump some of the salty fluid back into circulation and help reduce the swelling.

ARTHRITIS

Arthritis is a painful inflammation of one or more of the joints that "hinge" the body's bones.

What It Is

A joint is the meeting place of two bones. A soft, spongy material, called cartilage, provides cushioning where the bones meet. In the most common kind of arthritis, the cartilage is damaged and eventually disappears. This form of arthritis is called *osteoarthritis* or *degenerative arthritis*.

In *rheumatoid arthritis*, the second most common kind of arthritis, the membrane that lubricates the joint space becomes swollen and inflamed.

In another form of arthritis, called *gout*, the joint fluid is filled with sharp, microscopic crystals. This causes the joint to become red, hot, and very tender and swollen. Another form of arthritis is caused by an infection of the joint fluid with bacteria.

Over time, arthritis is not only painful but reduces the ability of the joint to move through its normal range of motion.

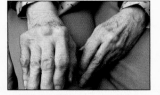

Arthritic hands.

Health Impact

Painful, less mobile joints can affect many of the simple pleasures and usual activities of daily life. Walking can become less safe and reduced mobility can contribute to falls. Arthritis that affects the hands can make cutting food, sewing, buttoning a button, and thousands of other "small" tasks difficult or even impossible. Aching joints can interfere with sleep. Additionally, the sudden development of a red, hot, and painful joint can be a medical emergency. For example, an *infection* of a joint can permanently damage the

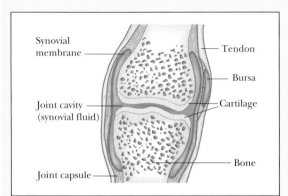

Normal configuration of joint structures.

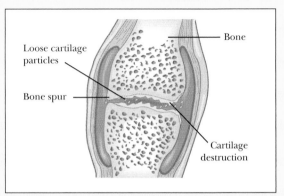

Osteoarthritis. Deterioration and deformity of joint structures from progressive destruction of cartilage and bone tissue.

joint in a matter of hours. Because most types of arthritis last a lifetime, strategies to live comfortably in spite of the arthritis are important.

VARIATIONS

Early Symptoms
- Swelling, redness, tenderness, and heat in the joints
- Stiffness, especially in the morning
- Fatigue
- Pain

Advanced Symptoms
- Bony deformity of the joints
- Limited joint movement
- Inability to walk or bear weight on a joint

ALERT

Black, tarry, and extremely foul-smelling stool can be a sign of internal bleeding from arthritis medicines. This needs to be reported to the doctor as soon as possible.

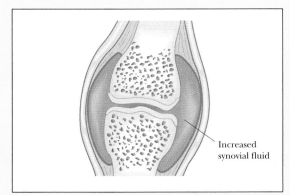

Increased synovial fluid

Rheumatoid arthritis. Inflammation affecting normal production of cushioning fluid.

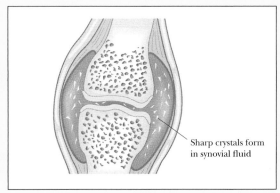

Sharp crystals form in synovial fluid

Gout. Acute inflammation with microscopic deposits in the joint fluid, swelling, and tenderness.

MEDICATION CHECKLIST

Analgesics. Analgesics are also called pain medications. For the mildest pain acetaminophen (Tylenol, among other brands) or aspirin (Bayer and other brands) commonly provide excellent relief. Pain medications that also reduce the inflammation of arthritis include the nonsteroidal anti-inflammatory drugs, or NSAIDs—aspirin in high doses, ibuprofen (Advil, Motrin, and others), naproxen (Naprosyn), indomethacin (Indocin), and many others. These drugs share side-effects that include causing stomach ulcers and ankle swelling. Narcotic pain medicines are occasionally used for more severe pain. The narcotics include acetaminophen with codeine (Tylenol and Codeine) and hydrocodone (Vicodin). They can cause constipation, drowsiness, and confusion.

Steroids. Steroids are used to treat the inflammation of certain types of arthritis. They can be injected into the joint or taken by mouth. Prednisone is the most common steroid taken by mouth. There are many side-effects that limit the use of these drugs.

Disease-Modifying Drugs. These drugs can actually prevent much of the joint destruction from certain types of arthritis. Methotrexate is a drug that requires frequent blood tests to make sure no problems are triggered by the drug. Others include hydroxychloroquine (Plaquenil).

Gout drugs. These drugs help treat or prevent gouty attacks. Common examples are colchicine, allopurinol (Zyloprim), and probenecid (Benamid).

YOUR ROLE

You can help your residents by making your facility as "arthritis friendly" as possible. For example, you can modify bathrooms and dining rooms to help these residents. Provide chairs with armrests to help residents safely transfer. Be aware that many arthritis drugs have side-effects, and familiarize yourself with the drugs your residents are taking. Also keep in mind that many people with arthritis have sudden attacks of worsening pain and swelling. Such a change in the resident's condition should be relayed to the doctor.

Medical Treatment
- Analgesics (pain medicines)
- Medication to reduce inflammation (for example, injections into the joints)
- Assistive devices, such as a cane or walker, to make walking and other daily activities easier
- Surgery to replace damaged joints

Residential Care Actions
- Make facility as fall safe as possible, with railings along hallways, banisters on stairs, and good lighting.
- Have modified utensils and tools for affected residents.
- Install elevated toilet seat with sturdy handrails.
- Remind residents to use assistive devices like canes and walkers when prescribed.
- Make entryways and doors wide enough to allow safe use of walkers and wheelchairs.
- Consider having a wheelchair available for residents who usually walk but are limited on long trips due to pain or slowness. This will allow easier access to doctor's offices, shopping, and recreational trips.

 DIET TIPS

- Provide extra fiber and fluids if constipation is present.
- Offer dietary supplements or small, frequent meals if appetite is poor.
- Many arthritis medicines cause less stomach pain when taken with food. If you are not sure when the medicines are to be given in relation to meals, ask the doctor.

FOR YOUR RECORDS

Health History
- Previous arthritis, gout attacks, ulcers, constipation
- Medication use
- Alcohol use

Current Needs
- Weight monitoring
- Monitoring functional status
- Monitoring for pain that keeps resident up at night
- Assistive devices

COMMON QUESTIONS

What causes arthritis?
Some forms of arthritis are clearly inherited, and some forms are caused by injury to a joint. Aging causes changes in joints that seem to make arthritis more likely to occur. Although some forms of arthritis are very common, not everyone develops arthritis as they age. In many cases, we do not yet have a good explanation as to why arthritis occurs.

Does diet affect arthritis?
Many major joints support our entire body weight when we walk or carry heavy things. If we weigh too much, the extra stress on the joint can cause excess wear and even speed up the arthritis process. The way diet affects arthritis most is when we eat too much and gain excess weight. Some forms of arthritis, such as gout and some cases of rheumatoid arthritis, do seem to respond to special diets, but this is best determined with the help of the doctor.

What level of activity is appropriate for the resident with arthritis?
During the peak of an arthritis attack, the painful joint might benefit from rest. The doctor may even prescribe a splint to allow the joint to rest. Most of the time, exercise is very helpful to keep the resident flexible and strong, and residents should stay as active as possible.

BLADDER PROBLEMS

Urinary incontinence is an involuntary loss of urine of sufficient frequency or severity to be a problem. It occurs in 15% to 30% of people over age 60 who live in the community, and in up to 50% of persons living in nursing homes. It accounts for over 10 billion dollars per year in health care expenditures in the United States. Other bladder problems are also common in the elderly. These range from the need to urinate very frequently, called *urinary frequency*, to the complete inability to pass urine at all, called *urinary retention*.

The urinary system.

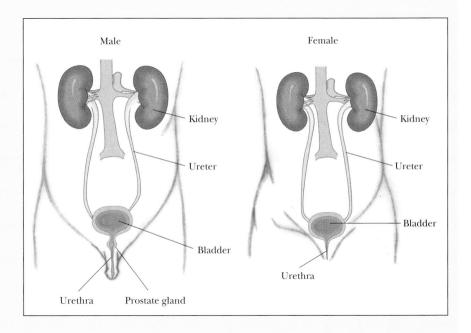

Male

Female

Kidney

Kidney

Ureter

Ureter

Bladder

Bladder

Urethra

Urethra   Prostate gland

What It Is

As we age, many factors change our bladder function. The lining of the bladder thins, and the tissues that support the bladder can become stretched and weakened. In men, the prostate gland enlarges and presses on the outlet of the bladder. Our defenses against infection weaken, and bladder infections are more common. Diseases are more common, as well, and many cause an increase in urination or a slowness of walking that increases the chance of accidental urination. Brain diseases, such as Alzheimer's disease, interfere with the mental ability to empty the bladder in a socially acceptable manner.

Health Impact   Incontinence of urine can be embarrassing, and many incontinent persons become isolated and depressed. Skin irritation and infection can occur when urine remains in contact with the skin. When the bladder cannot empty, severe pain can occur. If the urine is infected, bacteria can spread into the bloodstream and result in death.

The distance urine flows from the bladder to the urethra (where it is expelled) is much shorter in women than in men, and incontinence is twice as common in women than in men. Incontinence is a common reason for transferring a resident to a nursing facility. Even when it is manageable in a residential care facility, the added cost of laundry and incontinence garments is expensive and the social burden of embarrassment and isolation is great. Many cases of incontinence are completely treatable, and in most other cases the frequency can be decreased with medical treatment. Other bladder problems, such as urinary retention and urinary infection, are common problems in residents and your staff should be aware of them.

VARIATIONS

Urge Incontinence
- Leaking of urine associated with an intense urge to empty the bladder, frequency of urination, and only a very short warning before urine begins to flow
- May be worse in cold weather

- Leakage of urine with coughing, sneezing, lifting, or getting up from a sitting position
- Often only small quantities of urine leak out
- Tends to occur more often in women

Overflow Incontinence
- Almost continuous leakage or dribbling of urine, usually from a very full bladder
- Resident may be unaware of passing urine
- Often associated with prostate enlargement in men
- Frequently found in persons with neurological conditions such as multiple sclerosis and spinal cord diseases

Functional Incontinence
- Bladder function is usually normal
- Associated with mental confusion, severe depression, or physical conditions such as blindness or arthritis that prevents resident from reaching toilet in a timely fashion
- May be triggered by drugs that sedate the resident or create mental confusion

ALERT

Sudden development of incontinence might be a sign of a serious infection or stroke, and should be reported to the resident's doctor promptly.

MEDICATION CHECKLIST

Anticholinergic Drugs. These drugs are used to increase the time between the need to urinate, and are primarily used for urge incontinence. Some of them also have a direct action relaxing the bladder muscle. They all share side-effects of dry mouth, blurry vision, constipation and the risk of causing confusion. Common examples include propantheline (Probanthine), oxybutynin (Ditropan), Flavoxate (Urispas), and imipramine (Tofranil).

Cholinergic Drugs. These drugs increase the strength of the muscular contractions of the bladder, and are primarily used for overflow incontinence to improve poor bladder muscle function. They can cause side-effects of crampy abdominal pain and diarrhea. A commonly used drug in is bethanechol (Urocholine).

Estrogen Therapy. These drugs replace the hormones that are naturally produced by women prior to their menstrual periods stopping after menopause. After menopause, tissues of the bladder and urinary sphincter may become thin and dry, and giving estrogen in the form of pills, creams, or patches can lessen irritability of the bladder due to thin and dry tissues. Side-effects include vaginal bleeding, breast tenderness, and increased risk of certain cancers. These hormones are useful only for women and not for men. They are used to treat both urge and stress incontinence. Common examples include conjugated estrogen (Premarin) and estradiol (Estrace).

Nerve Transmitter Blocking Drugs. These drugs help relax the blockage of urinary flow that occurs from an enlarged prostate gland. They can prevent or lessen urinary retention, and they help decrease urinary frequency in some men with an irritated prostate gland. They are also used as blood pressure medications, and they can cause light-headedness and dizziness, especially if they lower blood pressure too much. Common examples include doxazosin (Cardura), terazosin (Hytrin), and prazocin (Minipres).

continued on following page

continued from previous page

Prostate Shrinking Drugs. Finesteride (Proscar) is a new drug that blocks the activity of the male sex hormone testosterone. Over time, it causes the prostate gland to shrink, and it is therefore useful when an enlarged gland causes urinary frequency.

Antibiotics. These are drugs used to kill the bacteria or yeasts that cause infections of the urine. Often, the new development of incontinence is due to an infection, and treating the infection can eliminate the incontinence. Many different antibiotics can be used—common examples include trimethaprim/sulfamethoxazole (Septra, Bactrim), ampicillin, norfloxacin (Norflox), ciprofloxacin (Cipro), and many others.

YOUR ROLE

You can do your residents a great service by making sure that incontinence is evaluated and treated by the resident's doctor. If you feel that the problem is not being taken seriously by the doctor, communicate your concerns and consider discussing a more thorough evaluation with the resident and his or her family. There are many special centers around the country to help those with incontinence. You might suggest referral to one of these centers if problems with incontinence are interfering with the resident's quality of life.

You can make your facility safer and better for people with bladder problems by installing grab rails and raised toilet seats to help them use the toilet more quickly and safely. Bathrooms should be well lit and the light switch readily available. For those residents who cannot make it quickly enough, consider bedside commodes or urinals within easy reach.

Train your staff to assist residents promptly when they ask for help reaching the bathroom, and explain to them that many residents just cannot "wait a minute" while they finish some other task. Have them report any change in urinary continence or signs of bladder infection or urinary retention. On some occasions, the doctor may ask your staff to keep an accurate record of the times the resident urinates and times when incontinence occurs. This type of voiding record can help the doctor diagnose and treat urinary problems.

Many confused elderly persons can be kept dry most of the time during the day if you regularly ask them to use the toilet, or even bring them to the toilet yourself. This works best if done as often as every two hours. You may learn the pattern an individual resident has—for example, some may need to urinate about half an hour after each meal. Demented residents may respond well to praise when they successfully empty their bladder in the toilet.

If a resident cannot be kept clean and odor-free, you should consider the possibility that your facility is inappropriate for that resident. Any breakdown of skin due to incontinence is a warning sign that the resident may need a higher level of care than your facility can provide.

Medical Treatment

- Confirming incontinence, retention or an infection with examination and testing.
- Treatment of urinary infections with antibiotics.
- Evaluation of the cause of incontinence and prescribing appropriate treatment (including medications, exercises, and surgery).
- Providing advice on incontinence skin care, incontinence garments, and improving availability of toileting (including bedside commodes and urinals).
- Urinary retention may require surgery or placement of a catheter into the bladder.

Residential Care Actions

- Given how common incontinence is and how embarrassing it can be, it is important to ask residents if they have problems with their bladder, or if they have trouble holding their urine.
- Notice any smell of urine on residents or their clothes, and report this to the doctor.
- Finally, because many causes of incontinence can be treated, be certain that any resident who has an incontinence problem receives an evaluation by the doctor for treatable causes.
- Make the bathroom as easily accessible and safe as possible.
- For residents who have mobility problems, consider switching their rooms closer to the bathroom or making commodes or urinals available in the room.
- For residents who need incontinence garments, such as adult diapers, help them have a ready supply.
- Any resident who develops increased frequency of urination, or complains of abdominal distention or pain on urination should be evaluated by his or her doctor.

DIET TIPS

- Restrict fluid after dinner only if approved by the doctor.
- Restrict sodium (salt) on doctor's orders, especially if resident has swollen ankles or other signs of congestive heart failure.
- Provide cranberry juice daily (can be sugar-free for diabetic or overweight residents) if urinary tract infections are common.
- Alcohol increases urination and should be avoided if incontinence is a problem.

FOR YOUR RECORDS

Health History

- History of bladder infections, incontinence, prostate problems, need to urinate frequently at night
- History of neurological conditions such as multiple sclerosis, stroke, Parkinson's disease, or Alzheimer's disease—all are associated with increased risk of bladder problems
- History of congestive heart failure, swollen ankles, diabetes—medical conditions which may be associated with increased need to urinate
- Medication use, especially diuretics
- Alcohol use

Current Needs

- Monitoring frequency and pattern of incontinence, waking up at night, frequent nighttime urination
- Reporting swelling of ankles to the doctor

COMMON QUESTIONS

Why would a person suddenly be unable to pass urine?
This problem most often occurs when there has been a gradual narrowing of the pathway from the bladder. Most commonly this is due to prostate enlargement in men, a mass pressing on the outlet of the bladder, or scarring of the passageway due to long-standing infection. Often an added factor is a medication that causes extra impairment of bladder emptying—nonprescription cold medicines or decongestants, antihistamines, and many pre-

scription medications. Severe constipation with hard stool forming a mass also can block flow from the bladder.

Should fluids be restricted in the evening to prevent the resident from needing to go to the bathroom at night?
This can sometimes be useful, but should only be done with permission from the resident's doctor. Dehydration is a serious problem in elderly persons, and therefore fluid restriction is often ill-advised.

When is a long-term urinary catheter needed?
Catheters are used for only a few situations. Sometimes the cause of obstructed urinary flow cannot be safely fixed, and a catheter is the best way to drain the bladder. At other times, the bladder does not adequately empty, and the resident is unwilling or unable to learn how to insert a clean catheter several times daily to drain the urine. Finally, sometimes skin ulcers on the buttocks cannot be kept clean and dry enough to heal without using a catheter. In general, catheters are not used simply for convenience, as serious complications are possible, including infection and bleeding from sores in the bladder and urethra.

When is surgery needed for incontinence?
When behavioral and drug therapies fail to provide satisfactory control of urination, there are surgical procedures that can give additional help. The bladder may need to be sewn internally to help support it, or the muscles that close the bladder outlet may need reinforcement. For men, surgery can treat the blockage of urine flow by an enlarged prostate gland.

Is there any dietary strategy that decreases urinary tract infections?
A glass of cranberry juice every day has been shown to decrease bladder infections!

BROKEN BONES

Broken bones, also called fractures, are just what they sound like—the bone is cracked, sometimes into separate pieces, and sometimes the crack is embedded in the bone.

What It Is

The injury to the bone may be due to a great force, such as a fall or car crash. Weakened bone, however, breaks from very minimal force. Symptoms may include:

- Pain in the affected area.
- Swelling and deformity of the affected area.
- Bruising around the area of pain.
- Instability at the area of injury.
- Occasionally, fragments of broken bone are visible through an area of injury.
- A bone may be broken even if nothing unusual is visible in the area of pain.

This is especially common in the elderly, whose bones are weakened by osteoporosis, the age-associated process that results in thin and brittle bones in many elderly people. This also causes certain types of fractures to be more common in the elderly.

Common Sites of Fractures in the Elderly

Upper arm/shoulder
Wrist
Pelvis
Hip
Knee
Back

Health Impact

Sharp fragments of broken bone can protrude from the skin or can cause severe bleeding internally. The broken area of bone can no longer function normally, and the whole area is likely to need to be kept perfectly still to allow healing. This means an operation or plaster cast for several weeks or months. The resident will need help with things that he or she usually can do independently, such as dressing or bathing. The plaster cast may be itchy, and the broken bone can remain painful. Certain broken bones, including many fractures of the spine, pelvis, and skull, are not treated with casts. These fractures are stable without a cast, and are treated simply by controlling pain by the use of medications and limiting painful activities.

For a young person who breaks a bone due to a major fall or car accident, the break means a prolonged healing process but usually an excellent recovery of full function. For an elderly person with thin bones that are brittle and break with minimal force, the first break can signal the start of a series of many broken bones, ultimately leading to poor function and increased disabilities. A broken hip can be catastrophic for an elderly person because many people die of complications of hip fractures. For example, a broken bone can lead to blood clots forming deep inside the leg, and these blood clots can break off and lodge in the lungs or heart, resulting in sudden death. The blood loss from a major broken bone can trigger a heart attack. About one fourth of elderly people who break a hip will never regain the ability to walk.

VARIATIONS

Closed Fracture
- Pain.
- Swelling can be at the site of the broken bone or below that area. For example, a fracture in the upper arm can cause swelling of the hand.
- Bruising.
- Deformity is often noted with fractures of arm or leg bones. The usually straight arm or leg will have a bend where there was not one before!

Open Fracture
- An open fracture is caused by a fragment of broken bone cutting through the skin surface. The broken bone can actually be seen sticking through the skin.
- Visible blood will often be evident where the skin is broken by an open fracture.
- Open fractures allow bacteria and dirt to enter the area of broken bone, and so are much more likely to get infected than simple fractures.

Potential Problems and Complications
- The swelling associated with a broken bone may compress nerves and blood vessels in a localized area of a limb. This causes increased numbness and pain, loss of muscle strength and often a purple discoloration in the limb beyond the area of compression. This condition is a medical emergency and requires immediately informing the physician.
- Broken bones that have healed improperly may never join or will join out of normal alignment.

- Many people experience pain or discomfort at the site of an old fracture during humid weather or when there is a change in the weather.

ALERT

Persistent pain after a fall or injury should be reported to the doctor as soon as possible. Any time a resident who usually walks loses that ability, contact the doctor as soon as possible.

MEDICATION CHECKLIST

Analgesics (Pain Medications). These drugs are used to treat the pain of broken bones. Common examples include acetaminophen with or without codeine (Tylenol, Tylenol and Codeine), and hydrocodone (Vidodin). Another family of pain medications commonly used are the nonsteroidal anti-inflammatory agents—aspirin, ibuprofen (Advil, Motrin), and many others.

YOUR ROLE

The best thing you can do for broken bones is to help prevent them by making your facility as "fall safe" as possible. Any resident who starts falling frequently needs evaluation because several "minor" falls may lead to a severe fall resulting in a fracture. When a resident returns to your facility after having a broken bone treated, determine if any additional help will be needed in daily activities such as dressing, toileting, and eating.

Medical Treatment
- Pain medicine
- Stabilizing the area of the broken bone to allow healing—often with a plaster cast
- Surgery, as needed, to put the broken bones together

Residential Care Actions
- Contact doctor immediately if an injury occurs and you are worried that a bone has been broken.
- Get information about how to care for injured area if doctor does not request immediate care.
- Ask for instructions on how to care for residents with a cast or sling from the doctor.

- Elevate the affected arm or leg if so instructed by the doctor.
- Inform the doctor if the resident develops skin problems or itching of the affected area.
- Be aware that resident may need additional assistance while broken bone is healing.

 DIET TIPS

- Dietary supplements or small, frequent meals if appetite is poor
- Supplemental calcium if recommended by the doctor
- Foods high in calcium such as milk or cheese if other dietary restrictions allow

FOR YOUR RECORDS

Health History
- Allergies
- History of constipation (many medicines used for pain can cause constipation)
- Medication use
- Alcohol use
- Description of events leading to injury

Current Needs
- Assistance and monitoring to help maintain functional status
- Assistive devices to perform activities of daily living
- Measures to relieve pain

COMMON QUESTIONS

How are you sure a bone is broken?
Although just looking at a badly broken bone can suggest it is broken, X-ray films are often needed to see if an injured area has a broken bone.

How long does a cast need to be on?
The doctor usually can give a good guess regarding how long a cast will be needed, but the doctor may need another X-ray evaluation before removing the cast to be sure the bone is healed.

What level of activity is appropriate for a resident with a broken bone?
Only the doctor can answer this. Be sure to ask before the resident returns to your facility.

Why do most fractures require a cast while a rib fracture does not?
Ribs need to move when we breathe. Tight binders restrict how deep a breath a person can take, and might lead to the development of pneumonia. Often the doctor treats a rib fracture with pain medicines and no binder or cast.

CANCER

Cancer is an uncontrolled growth of body tissue, which robs normal tissue of the nutrients and room it needs to function. Cancerous tissue also can spread into other, healthy tissue, and if untreated or if unresponsive to treatment, cancer can so damage the body's function that the person dies.

What It Is

Cells of the human body are continually replenished as old cells die and new cells are formed. This reproductive process is normally carefully controlled, and replacement cells look and function just like the cells they are replacing.

A cancer cell can differ from a normal cell in many ways, but of primary importance is the ability to "ignore" the body's signals to stop reproducing. A tumor may form that crowds normal tissues and prevents them from carrying out their essential functions. Or the cancerous cells may remain isolated, but because of their rapidly increasing number, may prevent a sufficient number of normal cells, such as red or white blood cells, to support normal body function.

Health Impact

A diagnosis of cancer can mean many things. Many cancers can be cured, so medical attention is needed. Some cancers cannot be cured, but treatment can prolong life and improve the quality of remaining life. Some cancers do not respond well to treatment, and thus goals of medical treatment emphasize quality of life instead of cure. This is a situation in which *hospice* care can be helpful.

Cancer also has an emotional effect, and even a minor and easily curable skin cancer can trigger sadness and even depression. More serious cancers frequently lead to depression at some time during the illness. The emotional aspects of cancer may require their own treatment, separate from the physical problems associated with the disease.

VARIATIONS

The stages to be expected in cancer depend on what type of cancer it is. The manner in which cancer affects the body, and therefore the signs and symptoms of disease, will depend on the type, location, and severity of the disease.

Warning Signs

The American Cancer Society has widely published a list of the Seven Early Warning Signs of Cancer. They can be remembered by the acronym CAUTION.

CAUTION

Change in bowel or bladder habits
A sore that does not heal
Unusual bleeding or discharge
Thickening or lump in breast or elsewhere
Indigestion or difficulty in swallowing
Obvious change in wart or mole
Nagging cough or hoarseness

Other Signs of Cancer that Should Trigger Concern

- Fatigue
- Weight loss
- Blood in the urine

Risk Factors

- History of previous cancer
- Family history of cancer
- Long-term exposure to carcinogenic substances, especially cigarette smoking, and environmental and industrial agents such as benzene, asbestos, uranium, coal tar, etc.
- Excessive exposure to X-rays or radiation
- Excessive exposure to sunlight
- High-fat and low-fiber diets

Most Common Cancers in the United States

Lung
Colorectal
Breast
Prostate
Uterus
Urinary tract
Mouth
Pancreas
Leukemia (blood)
Ovary
Melanoma (skin)

It should be noted that skin cancers are by far the most common cancers. Except for Melanoma, most skin cancers are very treatable and so rarely a cause of death.

ALERT

Learn the Seven Early Warning Signs of Cancer. If any of these symptoms are noticed, make sure the resident receives medical attention. Any resident receiving chemotherapy should be considered at high risk for other problems, because chemotherapy limits the body's ability to fight infections. Severe vomiting, chills, fever, or bruising in anyone receiving chemotherapy requires immediate medical attention.

MEDICATION CHECKLIST

Chemotherapy. Chemotherapy is a term used to describe drug therapy in cancer treatment. Different drugs are used to treat different cancers. If a resident is receiving chemotherapy, it is important to ask the doctor what to expect in terms of side-effects. It is very common for several anti-cancer drugs to be used together to maximize the chance of successful treatment.

Antinausea Drugs. These drugs help with the nausea that can occur in cancer or that can be a side-effect of chemotherapy. Common examples are prochlorperazine (Compazine) and trimethobenzamide (Tigan).

Analgesics. Analgesics, also called pain medications, are used to help reduce the pain that can occur with cancers. For minor pain, acetaminophen (Tylenol and others), aspirin, or ibuprofen (Advil and others) may be adequate. For more severe pain, narcotic analgesics such as codeine or morphine (MS Contin and others) can be used.

YOUR ROLE

Cancer is a chronic illness which will last for a long time. The resident must be helped to live with the illness and prescribed treatments. If the cancer progresses and it is known that the resident will not survive, the goal of care is to help control pain and promote as dignified a death as possible. You can help by providing emotional support and whatever physical help the resident needs. Remember that outside resources are available and guidance as well as support can be obtained from the local chapter of the American Cancer Society. You must also learn to recognize when the needs of the resident exceed the capacities of your facility and staff. In such circumstances, either extra help will need to be obtained or the resident will require transfer to a nursing or *hospice* facility.

Medical Treatment

- Anti-cancer drugs
- Radiation treatment
- Surgery
- Pain medication
- Oxygen

Residential Care Actions

- Weight monitoring.
- Monitoring pain or discomfort and effectiveness of pain medications.
- Transportation to radiation therapy or doctor.
- Helping to coordinate visits by nurses and other health professionals. Care during the final stages of an incurable cancer is sometimes provided by a special service called *hospice*. This type of service can often accommodate the resident staying at your facility by providing extra support for your staff and the resident's family as well as extra care and expertise for the resident.

 DIET TIPS

- Dietary supplements or small, frequent meals should be offered if appetite is poor.
- Certain anti-cancer drugs will require supplemental vitamins— ask the doctor.

FOR YOUR RECORDS

Health History
- Previous cancer
- Poor nutrition
- Medication use
- Functional status

Current Needs

Residents living with cancer can have a variety of special needs. These fall into the following categories:

- **Emotional.** Cancer can have a strong effect on self-image, sexuality, and mood. Depression is common and can respond to treatment.

- **Therapeutic.** This includes chemotherapy, surgery, radiation, biological therapies, laser treatment, and others. Generally one or several of these therapies are prescribed in an attempt to cure or at least slow the progression of the cancer.

- **Coping with treatment side-effects.** Unfortunately, each of the above-mentioned therapeutic approaches has its own set of side-effects that must be endured to allow treatment. Often the side-effects can be minimized with proper attention. Some of the side-effects may be permanent, such as the dry mouth and increased dental decay associated with radiation to the mouth. Under those circumstances, the doctor must help the resident cope with the effects of treatment.

- **Pain and symptom relief.** When a cancer cannot be cured, the next step is to minimize the discomfort or even pain associated with the remaining cancer. This might include pain medication, treatment for nausea, etc. This often can be performed without discharging the resident from your facility.

- **Ostomy care.** Surgical removal of all or a portion of the bowel or bladder leaves the resident with a new opening in the skin to drain the natural body excretions of urine or stool. To safely and cleanly handle these waste products, a bag is fastened to the skin to catch the bowel movements or urine. Residents with an ostomy require education to handle the skin care, sanitation, and appliances associated with an ostomy. Special nurses are often available to help with questions and to help the resident through the emotional aspects of this type of surgery.

- **Nutrition.** Cancer itself may be associated with impaired appetite, and a common side-effect of chemotherapy and radiation is loss of appetite and impaired sense of taste. Good nutrition is a key factor in fighting cancer and recovering from treatment. The special nutritional needs of each resident with cancer should be assessed and addressed.

COMMON QUESTIONS

How long can someone live with cancer?
Although cancer can and does kill, when treated successfully people can be cured or live for ten or more years with it. When cancer cannot be successfully treated, survival depends on the rate of growth of the cancer tissue as well as several other factors. At best, the doctor can sometimes give a rough estimate, but cannot accurately predict how long a person may live.

Should a resident be told he or she has cancer?
In general, people have the right to be informed of their diagnosis. Even if they are not directly told, they are likely to "figure it out." By trying to keep it a secret, you can actually create more fear and distress. Unfortunately, some families will try to insist that the nature of the illness be kept from a resident. This should be discussed with the doctor. A family conference with the doctor then may result in a decision to explain the diagnosis to the resident.

How much activity is appropriate for a person with cancer?
If the cancer is responding well to treatment, and the resident is feeling well, encourage full activity. If the resident is very weak or nauseated, clearly there will be a need to limit exertion. If a resident is physically strong but tends to stay in his or her room and not participate in daily activities, consider the possibility that depression is present and contact the doctor.

CONGESTIVE HEART FAILURE

A resident diagnosed with congestive heart failure suffers from a weakened heart muscle. The weakened heart can no longer function effectively in its role as a pump, thus the term "heart failure." Blood flow becomes sluggish, and the body's vital organs are affected. The kidneys, which normally eliminate excess salt and fluid from the body, now cause salt to be retained and extra fluids build up to dilute the extra salt. The body's tissues become "congested" with this extra fluid and may be noticed as swelling in the ankles and legs and in noisy, labored breathing.

What It Is

Congestive heart failure may result from a heart attack, damage caused by years of high blood pressure, or relatively rare diseases that affect the heart muscle itself. The weakness of the heart muscle progresses over time and can significantly shorten a person's life and reduce quality of life. However, with proper treatment, prognosis and quality of life can be improved.

Health Impact

The resident with congestive heart failure may experience a lack of energy and easy tiring resulting from insufficient blood flow to muscles. The resulting swelling in the bowels may interfere with appetite and cause constipation. Fluid in the lungs may cause mild or severe shortness of breath, difficulty breathing at night, impaired sleep and daytime sleepiness. Swelling of the ankles can cause discomfort, and dry, cracked skin on the legs that is easily infected.

VARIATIONS

Early Symptoms

- Ankle swelling
- Shortness of breath with exercise
- Cough
- Fatigue
- Weakness
- Increased urination at night

Advanced Symptoms

- Shortness of breath at rest
- Feeling of suffocation in the middle of the night
- Swelling of the legs and feet
- Loss of appetite
- Constipation

Potential Problems and Complications

- Kidney failure
- Sudden death

ALERT

Worsening of shortness of breath or increased swelling of legs needs to be reported to the doctor as soon as possible.

MEDICATION CHECKLIST

Diuretics. Commonly called "water pills," diuretics help rid the body of excess salt and water. They can limit the swelling of the legs and the collection of salty water in the lungs. Common examples include furosemide (Lasix), hydrochlorothiazide, and triamterene/hydrochlorothiazide (Dyazide or Maxzide).

Digoxin. This plant extract helps strengthen the heart and slow the heartbeat. Too much digoxin, however, can cause nausea or dangerously irregular heartbeats.

Vasodilators. These drugs expand the blood vessels, letting blood flow more easily and easing the heart's work. Examples include ACE inhibitors and hydralazine.

YOUR ROLE

Residents with congestive heart failure work with their doctor to achieve the proper balance between medication and salt restriction. If salt in the diet increases, or the heart suffers more damage, or if the medication requires adjustment, the person can get sick very quickly. By understanding this disease, you can look for early signs of trouble such as weight gain, increased swelling of the legs or ankles, or increased shortness of breath. Also, help make sure that the resident does not "cheat" on the diet by eating salty snacks.

Medical Treatment

- Medications to reduce water build up and improve heart function
- Oxygen

Residential Care Actions

- Sodium (salt) restricted diet, if prescribed
- Elastic stockings to improve blood flow in the legs, if doctor has ordered

- Elevating the legs to reduce swelling
- Regular weight checks to monitor fluid gains and losses
- Offering extra pillows to aid breathing during sleep
- Limiting alcohol use

 DIET TIPS

- Low sodium (salt) diet generally prescribed.
- Extra potassium in diet *only if prescribed*.
- Extra fiber if constipation present.
- Dietary supplements or small, frequent meals if appetite is poor.
- Alcohol use should be avoided.

FOR YOUR RECORDS

Health History
- History of heart attack
- History of high blood pressure
- Medication use
- Alcohol use

Current Needs
- Weight monitoring
- Adequate pillows for sleep
- Observation for and reporting of sleep disturbances
- Measures to help prevent or minimize urinary incontinence
- Assistance in maintaining functional status

COMMON QUESTIONS

How long can someone live with congestive heart failure?
Although congestive heart failure can and does kill, when treated successfully people can live for 10 or more years with it. When shortness of breath cannot be successfully treated, survival is often less than one year.

Why does the doctor not give enough of the water pill to completely get rid of the ankle swelling?
The water pills have their own side-effects, and using too much of them can lead to kidney failure or painful arthritis (called

gout). Using too much of the water pills can also result in light-headedness and fainting spells.

How much activity is appropriate for the resident with congestive heart failure?
Even short periods of inactivity can lead to a permanent loss of strength and balance. Residents should stay as active as possible.

CONSTIPATION

Constipation is the passage of hard, dry stool when attempting a bowel movement, or the build up of excessive amounts of stool in the bowel that interferes with normal function.

What It Is

Bowel movements result from the passage of waste products from our food that need to be eliminated from the body to promote good health. There is great variability among people in how often they need to move their bowels, and many people complain of constipation only because they have been taught or told that daily bowel movements are needed for good health. In fact, it may be perfectly adequate and healthy to move the bowels only every third day or so.

Constipation generally occurs when the natural contractions of the bowel are disturbed, so that the stool moves too slowly through the bowel. The bowel continues to absorb water from the stool, allowing dry and hard stool to form. Trouble occurs when the stool is so dry and hard that it causes pain on passage, or when so much stool builds up in the bowel that it presses on adjacent body parts, resulting in sores in the wall of the bowel or interference with bladder function. The build-up of stool also may cause a bloated feeling or reduce appetite.

Factors that slow the movement of stool include inadequate fluids, physical inactivity, and inadequate fiber in the diet. Medications can cause constipation, as well. Mentally impaired residents can experience constipation by resisting the urge to empty their bowels. Anything that causes pain on passing stool, like a sore in the rectal area, also can cause constipation, and overuse of laxatives or enemas can disturb the natural function of the bowel, leading to constipation. Certain diseases are particularly likely to cause constipation, including strokes, Parkinson's disease, and depression.

Health Impact

Dry, hard stool can press on the wall of the bowel so hard that ulcers or sores form, leading to bleeding that can potentially be life threatening. Hard "rocks" of stool can block normal flow in the bowel, letting only watery fluid pass while keeping most of the products of digestion blocked. This leads to the odd situation in which watery diarrhea passes, although the underlying problem is actually severe constipation. In extreme cases, such a large mass of stool builds up that the bladder, which is right in front of the rectum (storage area for stool) stops functioning. The urine then builds up, and painful distension of the bladder or incontinence (leakage of urine) can be the direct result of severe constipation.

VARIATIONS

Early Symptoms
- Decreased frequency of bowel movements
- Hard stools
- Difficulty passing stools
- Bloating
- Nausea
- Loss of appetite
- Distended abdomen

Potential Problems and Complications
- Blood from the rectum
- Fever
- Watery diarrhea
- Incontinence of stool or urine

ALERT

New incontinence of stool or urine, blood from the rectum, or distention of the abdomen needs to be reported to the doctor as soon as possible.

MEDICATION CHECKLIST

Dietary Fiber Supplements. Psyllium husks, bran, and other natural fibers can be added to the diet as a supplement. Other sources of supplementary fiber are available in tablets or in granular or powder form and can be sprinkled over salads or cereals or added to beverages. Common brands include Metamucil, Perdiem Fiber, Konsyl, Citrucel, Fiberall, FibrCon and Mitrolan.

Stool Softeners. Stool softeners hold water in the stool, helping to keep it soft. They usually contain salt and may need to be limited if the resident is on a low-salt diet. They only work if the resident drinks enough fluid. Common names include docusate (DSS, DOS Colace), and Surfak.

continued on following page

continued from previous page

Milk of Magnesia (MOM). This also carries water with it, and it often stimulates a bowel movement soon after it is taken.

Stimulant Laxatives. Stimulant laxatives use chemicals to irritate the bowel, and thereby stimulate a bowel movement soon after taken. If used regularly, they can damage the natural contractions of the bowel, making the resident even more constipated. Common types include senna, cascara, Dulcolax, Senekot, Carters Little Pill, and many more.

Enemas. An enema is the introduction of water, either tap water or salty water, into the rectum to soften the stool and stimulate a bowel movement. Some enemas are prepared with drugs that either stimulate the bowel or draw extra water into the bowel. A common brand is the Fleet enema, but many others are available, and plain warm water often works adequately.

Nonabsorbed Sugars. These forms of sugar are given as liquids. They can cause bloating and gas, but also help soften the stool and promote bowel movements. Common types include lactulose (Chronulac) and sorbitol.

YOUR ROLE

Any complaint of constipation should be communicated to the doctor if you believe the resident cannot mention the problem. You may find it helpful to write down a record of the resident's bowel movements for a week. Record the date of the bowel movements, the size, and any special characteristics like watery stools, hard stool, black or tar-like appearance, etc.

Unless instructed otherwise, encourage your residents to be physically active, to drink plenty of fluids (seven glasses of water per day), and to take plenty of natural fiber in their diet. Serve foods like fruits and vegetables. For residents who remain constipated after increasing the fluid and fiber quantities in their diet, discuss with their doctor the use of stool softeners, fiber supplements, laxatives, suppositories, and enemas. For some residents, you will be instructed to help them with enemas. Use only soft plastic or rubber tubes with side-openings, gently inserted in the anus after lubricating the anus with petroleum jelly or similar preparations. Never apply force or use a syringe, because perforation of the bowel can be dangerous. Use premeasured small-volume enemas such as a Fleet enema, or no more than 750 mL of warm water administered by enema bag.

Medical Treatment
- Stool softeners
- Increased water and other fluids in the diet
- Increased fiber in the diet
- Laxatives
- Suppositories
- Enemas

 DIET TIPS

- Offer extra fluid between meals as well as during meals.
- For extra fiber, substitute whole grain breads like wheat, rye, or pumpernickel for white bread. Try brown rice rather than white rice. Serve whole grain pastas and cereals. Bran can be substituted for bread crumbs in recipes. Dietary supplements of fiber can be given if doctor agrees.
- Prunes contain high amounts of magnesium and work very much like milk of magnesia.

FOR YOUR RECORDS

Health History
- Prior problems with constipation.
- Parkinson's disease, stroke, thyroid disease.
- Laxative use.
- Medication use.
- Chewing or swallowing problems can influence fiber and fluid intake.

Current Needs
- Monitoring usual frequency of bowel movements
- Adequate activity level and fluid intake

COMMON QUESTIONS

Is it necessary to have a bowel movement every day?
No, for many people less frequent bowel movements are perfectly healthy and acceptable.

How long should one wait for a bowel movement before getting concerned?
If pain, nausea, or other problems are present, the doctor should
be informed. If no bowel movement has occurred after four or
five days in a resident who usually has more frequent movements,
the doctor should be contacted. Everyone has a pattern that is
normal for them, and the key is that whenever there is a significant change in that pattern, the doctor should be notified.

Can poisons build up in the body if bowels don't move regularly?
No.

COUGH

A cough is the forceful exhalation of breath in response to an irritation in the lungs. It can be a sign of lung diseases such as asthma, cancer, bronchitis, or pneumonia. It can represent the body's response to irritants such as smoke or air pollution, or an allergic response to irritating pollens or dust.

What It Is

Cough is one way the body protects itself. For example, if a foreign body such as a food particle is inhaled into the lung, or "goes down the wrong pipe," a cough helps push the food particle out of the lung.

If an infection, such as pneumonia, tuberculosis, or bronchitis develops, cough helps rid the waste products, called *pus*, produced by the body's efforts to fight the infection. If this pus is coughed up, it forms *phlegm* (mucus) or *sputum*.

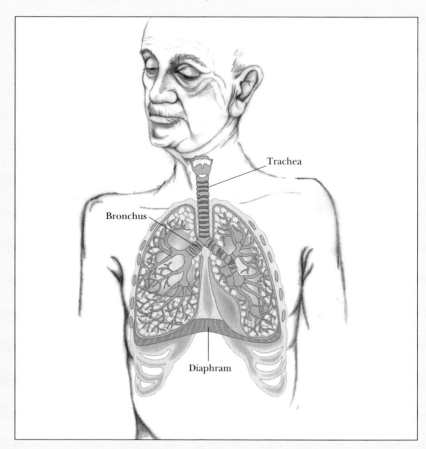

Trachea

Bronchus

Diaphram

Cough is a protective mechanism by which the body clears the respiratory tree of foreign substances.

Fluid that builds up in the lungs when the heart does not pump effectively (congestive heart failure) also causes cough. If the heart valves are narrowed or leaky, the lungs get stretched and cough occurs. Cough can be a side-effect of some medications, particularly the blood pressure medications called ACE inhibitors.

Health Impact

Coughing can be important in helping fight infections, but it can also be very annoying. Coughing can keep the resident (and others!) awake at night, and can spread certain infections. A new cough requires evaluation, particularly if it lasts longer than a few weeks. A chest X-ray test may be needed to diagnose and treat the problem.

Tuberculosis is particularly important in a residential care facility because it can spread easily among residents. A cough can be a warning that a tuberculosis infection has developed. Recognizing this allows treatment to begin before the disease spreads widely. Other infections of the lung can also cause coughing, and can spread among residents. Infections can be caused by viruses, fungus, and most commonly by bacteria. Such infections are called bronchitis if they involve the breathing tubes or *bronchi*, and pneumonia if the infection involves the deeper lung tissue.

VARIATIONS

Types of Coughs

- Dry, hacking, unproductive
- Productive, deep
- Annoying "tickle" in the throat

Associated Symptoms

- Fatigue
- Sleep impairment
- Stress incontinence (force of cough causes leakage of urine)
- Phlegm (mucos) production

Potential Problems and Complications

- Shortness of breath
- Loss of appetite
- Feeling of suffocation
- Fainting

ALERT

Worsening of symptoms, or new symptoms such as shortness of breath, should be reported to the doctor as soon as possible.

MEDICATION CHECKLIST

Cough Suppressants. These medications are often combined with other medicine that helps loosen phlegm and makes it easier to cough it up. Guaifenesin (Robitussin) is one of these medications and may be combined with narcotics to suppress cough, such as codeine or dextromethorphan (Robitussin DM). A pill used to relieve cough is benzonatate (Tessalon Perles).

Antibiotics. Antibiotics are used to fight infections that cause cough. Common examples include tetracycline, erythromycin, trimethoprim/sulfa (Septra or Bactrim), and others.

Bronchodilators. Bronchodilators are drugs that help expand the breathing tubes in the lungs, thereby making it easier to breathe. However, some have the side-effect of making the heart beat too fast, especially when used in excess. Although bronchodilators can be prescribed in pill form, most often they are prescribed for use in an inhaler (commonly called a "puffer"). Common examples include albuterol (Ventolin, Proventil) and ipratropium (Atrovent).

Steroids. Steroids are drugs that reduce inflammation in the breathing tubes of the lungs. Although they can be prescribed in pill form (most often as prednisone), more often they are prescribed for use in an inhaler. Common examples include triamcinolone (Azmacort), flunisolide (AeroBid), and beclomethasone (Beclovent, Vanceril).

Diuretics. Diuretics, also called water pills, actually help rid the body of excess salt *and* water. They can also limit the collection of salty water in the lungs if the cough is due to congestive heart failure. Common examples include furosemide (Lasix), hydrochlorothiazide, and triamterene/hydrochlorothiazide (Dyazide).

YOUR ROLE

Cough should be treated as a warning, and you should help a resident who has a new cough obtain medical attention to identify the cause of the cough. In many cases, a virus could be spreading through your facility, with many residents getting cough and cold symptoms at the same time. In such cases, you may discuss the problem with the doctor over the phone and obtain a prescription for a cough suppressant. Any resident with a cough who develops other problems such as shortness of breath or fever should be evaluated by the doctor.

Medical Treatment

- Cough suppressants including cough syrups
- Antibiotics to fight infection
- Inhalers (puffers) to improve breathing
- Chest X-ray evaluation
- Diuretics (water pills) if cough is due to fluid in the lungs
- Oxygen
- Hospitalization to treat serious problems

Residential Care Actions

- Sodium (salt) restricted diet if prescribed by doctor for resident with congestive heart failure
- Supervision of medication and oxygen use
- Discouraging cigarette smoking
- Regular tuberculosis testing (skin tests or X-ray evaluation)

 DIET TIPS

- Low-sodium (salt) diet if prescribed by doctor
- Extra fluids if phlegm is hard to bring up or is very dry and sticky
- Extra fiber and fluids if cough suppressants with codeine or dextromethorphan are being used
- Dietary supplements or small, frequent meals if appetite is poor

FOR YOUR RECORDS

Health History

- Previous lung disease
- Congestive heart failure
- Previous stroke or other problems that make swallowing difficult
- Medication use
- Smoking history
- Results of tuberculosis screening

Current Needs
- Residents with chronic cough should have adequate facial tissues available to discourage them from spitting phlegm.
- Fluids (juices, water) should be offered frequently to help the resident cough up any dry, sticky phlegm.

COMMON QUESTIONS

Our facility requires tuberculosis testing for each resident at the time of admission. Does testing need to be repeated?
Although regulations differ from state to state, the medical reasons to check regularly are the same everywhere. Tuberculosis is quite common in residents in residential care, and it can spread quickly. The use of a yearly tuberculosis test is to see if there is an unknown infection that may be spreading "silently." It can be very useful to require a skin test every year to help prevent unpleasant surprises. This must be ordered by a doctor. The skin testing can be administered by a nurse.

Why does the doctor not keep the resident on cough medicine indefinitely?
Cough medicine can have side-effects and may not work in a particular resident. Some residents who have permanent damage to their lungs may always have some coughing, and medicines are saved for situations in which the cough is especially severe. In particular, the narcotics that are used to decrease coughing can be constipating.

The resident's cough is still a problem, but the antibiotic the doctor prescribed has run out. What should I do?
Even after the infection of pneumonia or bronchitis is treated, the cough may persist. It should slowly decrease over a period of weeks. If it is not getting better, or persists longer than a few weeks, let the doctor know.

Dementia

Dementia means loss of mental abilities as a result of a disease process or illness.

What It Is

Dementia is different from mental retardation, in which mental abilities have been impaired since birth. Dementia usually starts with a loss of recent memory and an impaired ability to learn new information.

Any disease that damages the brain can cause dementia. The most common disease is Alzheimer's disease. This condition is at least in part inherited, but there is still much to learn about the cause and treatment. Another common cause of dementia is the brain damage caused over time by many small strokes; this is called *multiple infarction dementia*. Multiple infarction dementia is usually found in people who have had high blood pressure or diabetes for many years. Alcoholic dementia is caused by years of drinking too much alcohol. There are dozens of other diseases known to cause dementia.

Health Impact

As the disease progresses, the person with dementia loses the ability to speak easily and to understand the speech of others. Ability to perform complicated activities like driving, balancing a checkbook, or working may be lost, and eventually the individual loses the ability to accomplish simple tasks like dressing, bathing, or even eating.

Poor memory and judgment means a person with dementia needs help. When dementia is mild in severity, simple reminders to change clothes, eat regularly, and bathe may be enough. As the dementia progresses, the resident will need help such as financial supervision, help picking out clothes, cutting food, and so forth. Severe dementia may mean the resident needs more help than you can safely provide, and other living arrangements may need to be found.

VARIATIONS

Early Symptoms

- Poor recent memory
- Increasing forgetfulness

- Extra sensitivity to sleeping pills and other sedating drugs
- Confusion when ill or in a new environment
- Change in personality
- Poor judgment. Makes resident subject to injury as when he or she tries to balance on a rickety step stool, or subject to financial abuse as when unscrupulous or fraudulent salespersons sell them unnecessary items

Progressive Symptoms

- Poor understanding of daily events, due to poor memory and difficulty understanding complex events
- Forgetting important information
- Losing personal items
- Forgetting to bathe or change clothes
- Difficulty with tasks such as dressing
- More frequent episodes of confusion
- Waking up at night confused

Advanced Symptoms

- Forgetting who family members are
- Difficulty talking or understanding speech
- Forgetting how to cut food or feed one's self
- Problem behaviors such as pacing, chanting, refusal to bathe, hitting other residents, etc.
- Hallucinations
- Seizures

ALERT

Worsening of confusion or change in functional status needs to be reported to the doctor as soon as possible. Remember that the resident may not complain and may be unable to explain exactly what is bothering him or her. You must always be on guard for changes that might signal an important new problem.

MEDICATION CHECKLIST

Tacrine (Cognex). This is the only drug approved to treat the memory loss of mild to moderately severe dementia. The effect of this drug is a slight improvement or slower decline in mental ability rather than a dramatic improvement. While a resident is being treated with this drug, he or she will require regular blood tests to help avoid damage to the liver.

continued on following page

continued from previous page

Antipsychotic Drugs. These drugs help diminish the hallucinations or confused thoughts that sometimes occur with dementia. They both decrease the frequency of hallucinations and delusions and decrease the severity of those problems that remain. Examples are haloperidol (Haldol) and thioridazine (Mellaril). Side-effects like a stiff gait and lip-smacking movements make these drugs best used only when absolutely necessary.

Antianxiety Drugs. These drugs help calm the fear that often occurs in dementia residents when they do not understand what is being done to them. They can be useful to calm the resident prior to a bath or dental visit. Examples are oxazepam (Serax) or lorazepam (Ativan). Another type of antianxiety drug such as buspirone (Buspar) can be used regularly to calm nervousness that results in refusal to cooperate with necessary care.

Note: The use of sedatives and antipsychotic drugs is known as "chemical restraint" when doses are high enough to cause sedation, rigidity, or other serious side-effects. Such use of medication is considered poor medical care. However, the same drugs are used safely and appropriately in lower doses for treating delusions, hallucinations, paranoia, or anxiety that interferes with the resident's quality of life.

YOUR ROLE

Residents with dementia require careful supervision for simple tasks and display poor judgment and safety awareness as part of their illness. Your responsibility in caring for them is to make your facility as safe as possible. Caring for them in this respect is similar to caring for young children. Simple precautions like making sure the hot water from the faucet cannot cause a burn will help prevent injury. Putting alarms on doors can prevent residents from wandering outside and injuring themselves. Observe to see that the resident does not eat non-food items that can cause harm. Monitor appetite and bowel movements, and look for any unusual signs that might be an early warning of additional medical problems.

Another important problem to be sensitive to is withdrawal or depression. If a resident stops participating in social activities, inform family members or the doctor. If you care for many residents with dementia, read and learn as much as you can about the condition. Consider joining your local chapter of the Alzheimer's

Association to take advantage of their publications, educational programs, and general expertise.

Medical Treatment
- Testing to see if the dementia has a treatable cause
- Drugs to help improve memory
- Drugs to improve problem behaviors that sometimes accompany dementia

 DIET TIPS

- Food should be simple to eat (offer plenty of finger foods).
- Offer juice or other beverages between meals.
- Offer dietary supplements or small, frequent meals if appetite is poor.
- Alcohol use should be avoided.

FOR YOUR RECORDS

Health History
- Alcohol use
- High blood pressure; previous strokes
- Medication use
- Episodes of wandering; violence or injury to others
- Tobacco use
- Wakeful pattern at night
- Urinary or fecal incontinence

Current Needs
- Reminders and supervision of daily activities.
- Protection from abuse (physical, emotional, financial).
- Observation for signs of worsening confusion or other changes in the resident's condition.
- Weight monitoring to look for change in weight. Dementia residents can lose weight due to depression or difficulty feeding themselves or even swallowing, or they may gain weight due to forgetting they have eaten and therefore eating again.
- Use of community resources such as adult day care centers.

COMMON QUESTIONS

How long can someone live with dementia?
Although dementia can progress to starvation and death, usually

death results from some other process, such as pneumonia. Some dementias progress very slowly, and the resident may not exhibit signs for many years. Other dementias progress rapidly and the resident will need placement in a nursing facility within a year or so of needing residential care. After the ability to eat is lost, artificial feeding through a feeding tube must be started or the person will lose weight rapidly and then be unable to fight infection such as pneumonia or a bladder infection, and death may result.

When is dementia too severe to be cared for in a residential care facility? In general, this will depend on your particular facility. Severely demented individuals need personal care such as feeding, constant supervision, and assistance getting out in case of fire or other disaster. Some residential care facilities are prepared to provide such intensive services, while others are not. If a resident poses a danger to others or interferes with their care, then something must be done to change these behaviors or the resident will need to be transferred to a facility that can handle such residents.

What are some non-drug measures that can help with problem behaviors in residents with dementia?
Having a poor memory can be very frightening, and having someone take your clothes off and put you in the shower can be terrifying for a resident with dementia. It is always wise to explain who you are and what you are doing, to help relieve the fear and anxiety that can lead to violent behaviors. It helps for the resident to be able to see and hear well to minimize fear. Always check to be certain that hearing aids are functioning and inserted properly and that glasses are worn. Calm music, quiet environments, and diverting activities help avoid some problem behaviors. If two residents start arguing, try to separate them and then distract them; soon they are likely to forget what it was that they were fighting over!

What types of activities are appropriate for the resident with dementia?
Activities that are easily understood and are non-threatening—playing catch with a large ball, working with clay or non-toxic paints, listening to music, or singing familiar songs are just a few suitable activities. Many communities have special day centers for individuals with dementia.

DIABETES

Diabetes is a disease in which the ability of the body to control the level of sugar in the blood is impaired. Many people refer to the disease as *sugar diabetes*, but its proper name is *diabetes mellitus.*

What It Is

The body's blood supplies essential nutrients and other substances to all body cells. These substances are normally maintained in proper amounts by various control mechanisms. Sugar levels are controlled primarily by a hormone called insulin which is produced in the pancreas.

Sugar is a substance that must be carefully controlled, because even though it is an important source of fuel, too much sugar in the blood over a period of many years can cause organ damage, poor circulation, and increased risk of infection.

Abrupt changes in blood sugar level—for example, a sudden drop or dramatic increase—also can permit serious problems to develop over a short period of time, and a resident with diabetes is at risk of a condition called *diabetic coma.*

Health Impact

Diabetes is often "silent," meaning there may be very few symptoms until serious damage has been done. Serious health problems can be prevented only by carefully monitoring blood sugar, and then controlling the high blood sugar with treatment.

However, infections and other medical problems can cause a sudden loss of control over blood sugar in a resident who is normally doing well. In a diabetic resident, the first sign of pneumonia or a bladder infection might be the problems you would otherwise associate with very high blood sugar (thirst, frequent urination, or even mental confusion).

An additional problem in managing diabetes is that sometimes the treatment works too well! If the diabetes medication or insulin lowers the blood sugar too much, the brain and other organs will not receive enough fuel. This can cause headache, difficulty concentrating, or even fainting.

VARIATIONS

Classic Symptoms

- Thirst
- Frequent urination

- Lack of energy
- Poor healing of cuts or other injuries
- Numbness of fingers or toes

Signs of High Blood Sugar

- Excessive thirst and urination
- Vaginal itching or white discharge
- Blurry vision
- Sleepiness or loss of alertness

Signs of Low Blood Sugar

- Difficulty concentrating
- Mental confusion
- Bizarre behavior
- Rapid heartbeat, sweaty palms, nervousness

Potential Problems and Complications

- Blindness
- Poor circulation in legs; amputation
- Stroke
- Heart attack
- Kidney failure

ALERT

Sometimes a resident's medication can lower blood sugar too much, especially if the resident has had a poor appetite. At other times, an infection or other medical illness can cause blood sugar to get very high. Both conditions can cause confusion or other changes in brain function. The doctor must be informed of any change in alertness or mental functioning.

MEDICATION CHECKLIST

Oral Hypoglycemic Drugs. Commonly called "diabetes pills," these drugs help the body burn sugar more efficiently. The risk associated with their use is that if the resident does not eat properly, the blood sugar can become dangerously low. Common examples include glipizide (Glucatrol), glyburide (Glynase), and tolazamide (Tolinase). Sometimes another medication, called metformin (Glucophage), is used by itself or added to insulin or another oral medication. This medication must not be given if a resident suddenly becomes ill, because it can cause problems if a resident becomes dehydrated or develops kidney failure.

continued on following page

continued from previous page

Insulin. The insulin used to treat diabetes is a substitute for the body's own insulin. It must be injected to be effective. It is available in both short- and long-acting forms and in combination forms. The short-acting form is called *regular insulin*; a common long-acting form is called NPH insulin. Mixtures of 70:30 and 50:50 of NPH and regular insulin are commonly used.

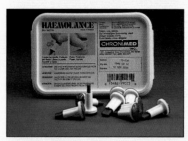
finger-stick device

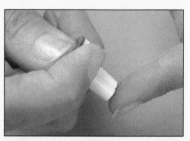
finger-stick technique

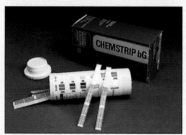
blood glucose strips

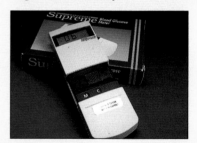
glucose monitor

YOUR ROLE

Diabetic residents can forget or refuse to take medication and may not adhere to their diet, because they do not "feel" the high blood sugar. They need to be encouraged to comply with treatment. Some people with diabetes are prescribed instruments to help check blood sugar regularly. You should encourage use of these instruments, and help the resident keep a record of blood sugar levels to help the doctor adjust treatment as needed. If possible, learn how to use the blood sugar testing instruments, so you can help as needed.

Numbness of the feet can increase the risk of minor cuts or sores developing into serious problems. The resident needs regular attention from a foot doctor (podiatrist). This can be made easier if you can arrange for a podiatrist to make regular visits to your facility.

Understand the signs that may be seen when blood sugar is too low or too high. Have some juice or candy available to give the resident quickly if signs of low blood sugar develop. This can be life-saving when blood sugar is low, and will not be particularly dangerous if the blood sugar is too high instead. If symptoms persist after a few minutes, call the doctor, because problems with low blood sugar usually respond quickly to some juice or candy. Signs of high blood sugar generally require informing the doctor, as some adjustment of the resident's medication may be needed. Very high blood sugar may be a sign that an infection is present and often requires transferring the resident to a hospital emergency room for further evaluation.

Medical Treatment

- Diet and lifestyle counseling
- Exercise
- Monitoring blood sugar
- Oral diabetes medications
- Insulin injections
- Regular podiatry and ophthalmology care

Residential Care Actions

- Calorie- or fat-restricted diet
- Weight monitoring
- Support for resident who is trying to stop smoking
- Limit alcohol use
- Monitor medication use
- Report any evidence of medication side-effects

 DIET TIPS

- A low-fat diet is generally prescribed by the doctor, because problems associated with fatty deposits in the blood vessels (stroke and heart attack) are among the most serious problems that can result from diabetes.
- Decreasing the sugar in the diet is usually considered less important, but eliminating sugary sweets is often prescribed by the doctor.
- Extra fiber in the diet can improve control of blood sugar and improve bowel function.
- Alcohol use should be avoided or kept within recommendations of doctor if allowed.

FOR YOUR RECORDS

Health History
- Previous stroke, heart attack, or kidney failure
- High blood pressure
- Previous problems with very high or very low blood sugar
- History of smoking
- Medication use
- Alcohol use

Current Needs
- Weight monitoring.
- Recent blood sugar values and "target" values.
- Dietary recommendations and prohibitions.
- Skin care.
- Foot care.
- Packets of table sugar or candy to treat signs of low blood sugar.
- Exercise.
- If resident self-monitors blood sugar, he or she will need space to store and clean equipment and will regularly need test strips and alcohol swabs.

COMMON QUESTIONS

Why should a resident take medication that may be expensive or cause side-effects when there are no symptoms of diabetes?
There is excellent evidence that treating high blood sugar from diabetes can prevent strokes, heart failure, and premature death. After problems develop it may be too late to obtain good results from treatment.

Why is it that all diabetics cannot take oral medication for it? Why do some need to inject insulin?
There are different causes of diabetes, and different treatments work better for each type. Some diabetics have lost their ability to produce insulin. They are likely to need injected insulin as a treatment. Other diabetics make plenty of insulin, but the insulin fails to have its usual effect in lowering blood sugar. For these diabetics, losing weight sometimes will control the disease. If diet alone fails to control diabetes, an oral medication is likely to help. If one medication fails, another medication may be added or tried alone, or the resident may be switched to insulin.

What level of activity is appropriate for the diabetic resident?
Physical activity can help lower blood sugar and improve control of the resident's diabetes. Exercise should be encouraged. If heart disease is present or you have other questions, discuss specific recommendations with the doctor.

DIARRHEA

Diarrhea is an increase in the frequency of bowel movements and a change in consistency of the stool from solid to liquid.

What It Is

An important function of the bowel is to absorb water from waste material, or stool, as it passes through the digestive tract. When this function is interfered with by disease, diarrhea may result. Diarrhea stools are soft and watery, and the number of bowel movements per day can be markedly increased.

Diarrhea can be caused by infections, and the infection can spread by contact with the loose stool. Food can be contaminated with bacteria or other substances, and the resulting diarrhea can be a form of food poisoning. Diseases of the bowel, such as cancer, can cause diarrhea. It can also be a side-effect of drugs. Excessive use of stool softeners or antacids are common drug-related causes of diarrhea. Antibiotics also can cause diarrhea by killing some of the normal bacteria that live in the bowel. Certain foods can cause diarrhea in susceptible persons if taken in large quantities. For example, elderly persons may be sensitive to milk and milk products, and will develop diarrhea if too much milk is in the diet. Severe constipation can also lead to diarrhea, because "rock hard" stool can block the bowel, letting only watery fluid pass.

Health Impact

Diarrhea can cause so much fluid loss that the resident becomes dehydrated. This can lead to light-headedness, dizziness, or even fainting. Normal body salts are lost in diarrhea stools, and loss of these salts can cause weakness and an irregular heartbeat. The stool may be irritating to the skin, causing rashes or skin ulcers. Additionally, diarrhea can be socially embarrassing, causing the resident to become withdrawn and isolated.

VARIATIONS

Primary Symptoms

- Frequent, loose, watery stools
- Increased frequency of bowel movements
- Weakness, light-headedness
- New incontinence of stool

Associated Symptoms

- Loss of appetite
- Dry mouth
- Weakness
- Dizziness

Potential Problems and Complications

- Dehydration
- Low blood pressure
- Kidney failure
- Death

ALERT

Most diarrhea caused by infection and food contamination lasts only a day or so and then stops. Diarrhea that lasts more than two days or is accompanied by blood in the stool may mean a drug-related problem or underlying bowel disease that will require the doctor's attention.

If food poisoning is suspected, it may be important to contact the local department of health to investigate, because future cases may be prevented by identifying problems in the handling or storage of food. It is in your interest to do so, because it will show a clear effort on your part to prevent this type of problem.

MEDICATION CHECKLIST

Antidiarrheal Drugs. These drugs slow the activity of the bowels and can relieve the diarrhea. Common examples are loperamide (Imodium) and diphenoxylate (Lomotil). Other drugs add bulk to the stool and can help with diarrhea. An example is attapulgite (Kaopectate).

Antibiotics. Antibiotics can kill the bacteria that cause some types of diarrhea. Many different antibiotics are used for this purpose.

Electrolyte Replacement Solutions. These drinks are used to replace the salts and water that are lost with diarrhea. Many sport drinks, such as Gatorade can be used. It should be noted that many of these drinks contain sugar and should be used with caution in diabetics.

YOUR ROLE

Make sure that food is properly stored and handled in your facility. Teach staff to wash hands between interactions with residents, and particularly after caring for residents with diarrhea. Consider food poisoning whenever there are several residents with vomiting, diarrhea, or abdominal pain at the same time. When a resident has diarrhea, carefully observe for signs of dehydration, such as a change in alertness, weakness, or light-headedness, which should be reported to the doctor. Any diarrhea that persists for more than two days or that begins after a new medication is started should be reported.

Medical Treatment

- Fluid replacement (either by mouth or by intravenous fluid)
- Medication to treat the cause of the diarrhea
- Medication to slow or stop the diarrhea

Residential Care Actions

- Special diet, as prescribed by doctor.
- Encourage fluids.
- Careful observation.
- Bedside commode.
- Supervise medication.
- Contact doctor if condition changes or diarrhea persists.
- If several residents develop diarrhea at the same time, consider the possibility of food poisoning or flu. If in doubt ask the doctor for advice.
- Make sure the hygiene practices of your facility minimize the risk of spreading diarrhea from one resident to another.
- Make sure food preparation and serving practices of your facility minimize the risk of food poisoning.

 DIET TIPS

- Obtain advice from the resident's doctor regarding any dietary changes that may be recommended until the diarrhea stops.
- Be certain that food is properly stored, cooked to appropriate temperatures, and promptly served.
- Extra fiber and fluids should be offered if constipation is usually present.
- Alcohol use should be avoided.

FOR YOUR RECORDS

Health History
- Previous episodes of diarrhea
- Previous episodes of constipation
- Medication use
- Alcohol use

Current Needs
- Is there a history of milk or milk products causing diarrhea? If so, such items may need to be avoided.
- Are occasional problems with diarrhea a well-known problem with this resident? If so, consider asking the doctor if a drug such as Imodium can be available and used without having to call the doctor each time.
- Certain medications should be "held" and not given to the resident if diarrhea is occuring. One diabetes medication, metformin (Glucophage), can be very dangerous if the resident gets dehydrated. Ask the doctor if there is any special way of handling other medications if diarrhea develops.

COMMON QUESTIONS

What is the best food to eat when a person has diarrhea?
Easy-to-digest food is best to start with, such as toast, rice, applesauce, and so forth. Liquids are very important, and often ginger ale that has been opened to let the bubbles disappear is easy on the stomach.

This resident is always constipated. Why has diarrhea suddenly developed?
Although constipated residents can develop food poisoning or any of the other causes of diarrhea, severe constipation can result in another problem called *fecal impaction*. In this situation, "rock hard" stool forms a ball in the bowel and blocks the passage of normal stool. Only watery liquid stool can pass, making it seem that diarrhea is the problem when really the underlying problem is severe constipation. The treatment for this diarrhea might even be enemas.

Several of our residents have diarrhea. How can we be sure it is not food poisoning?
Although it might not be possible to be completely sure, a good clue would be if all affected residents ate the same food, while those who skipped a particular dish were spared the diarrhea.

FALLS

Falling is common among the elderly, and although most falls do not result in injury, some can result in bruises, sprains, or broken bones. Many falls are preventable, and each fall should be considered a warning—the next fall could possibly cause a major injury, resulting in loss of independence and transfer to a different care facility.

What It Is

A fall results from an unintended loss of balance while standing, sitting, or transferring to or from a bed, chair, toilet, or bath. Some falls are truly due to chance, when one resident accidentally pushes another resident or a handrail breaks while supporting a resident. Other falls are much more predictable, because they result from weakness or other physical problems. The following specific factors predispose residents to falls.

- Muscle weakness.
- Disease states such as stroke.
- Parkinson's disease and other movement disorders.
- Drugs, especially if a medication makes a resident sleepy, light-headed, or dizzy. Even water pills can cause a fall by making the resident have to hurry to get to the bathroom. Alcohol and sleeping pills can also lead to falls.
- Sudden illnesses like pneumonia or bladder infections can trigger a fall. The illness impairs balance from factors such as dehydration, fever, and mental confusion. Urinary urgency from a bladder infection may cause rushing to the bathroom and an associated fall.
- Fainting or seizures.
- Environmental factors (poor visibility; bathrooms located too far from the bedroom; exposed electrical cords or frayed rugs).

Health Impact

Obviously falls can cause serious physical injuries, including potentially fatal hip fractures. Other symptoms may include.

- Bruises
- Cuts
- Broken bones
- Decreased willingness or ability to walk
- Depression

Other consequences of falls are not necessarily visible, but result in prolonged pain. Some of the saddest results of falls are the changes in lifestyle that a resident may impose on himself or herself after a fall, such as reluctance to participate in activities or to leave the facility. In some cases, a resident may "take to bed" or become very depressed.

It is estimated that the average person over age 65 falls twice a year. Falls are the leading cause of accidental death and the seventh leading overall cause of death in persons over age 65. The cost of fall-related injuries exceeds $7 billion annually.

Given the relatively brittle bones of older people, a fall is much more likely to result in an injury for an older person than for a younger one. Usually, several non-injury falls occur before a serious injury occurs. If a fall with no injury occurs, use the fall as an opportunity to find treatable causes of the fall and prevent future falls.

VARIATIONS

Minor Falls
- No injury.
- Minor injuries—bruises, cuts, etc.
- Often there is a loss of confidence and willingness to walk after a minor fall.

Major Falls
- Broken bones
- Sprains, torn ligaments, other major injuries
- Restriction of activity
- Loss of safety in residential care

ALERT

Any fall needs to be reported to the doctor, but falls in which injuries occur need to be reported as soon as possible. Non-injury falls can be reported at a regular doctor visit.

MEDICATION CHECKLIST

Medications are more often the cause of a fall than a treatment. Therefore, often the best thing to do after a fall is to talk to the resident's doctor who can determine if any medications can be stopped.

YOUR ROLE

Falls are a major problem in residential care, and are frequently the cause of transfer to the hospital or into a nursing facility. Falls can be prevented in many cases, and you can help by making your facility as safe as possible for all residents. If a resident falls frequently, you can help the doctor by discussing the change in the resident's condition and noting the circumstances of falls as carefully as possible.

Medical Treatment
- Treatment of cuts, sprains, and broken bones
- Medication for any pain and swelling
- Prescription of canes, walkers, or wheelchairs
- Identifying factors that contribute to the fall and measures to help prevent future falls

 DIET TIPS

- Weight loss and muscle weakness are important causes of falls. Dietary supplements or small, frequent meals should be offered if resident is weak or losing weight.
- Alcohol use should be avoided.

FOR YOUR RECORDS

Health History
- Previous falls, injuries, fainting
- Recent weight loss
- Previous stroke
- Parkinson's disease or other movement disorders
- Medication use
- Alcohol use

Current Needs
- Extra safety precautions
- Improved lighting
- Removing exposed electrical cords and loose rug edges
- Installing or securing handrails, especially in bathrooms
- Reporting any change in resident alertness or other conditions
- Use of cane or walker
- Measures to help prevent or manage urinary or fecal incontinence

COMMON QUESTIONS

Why should it be my responsibility to prevent falls?
Accidents can be prevented. If there are things that your facility or staff could have done to prevent a fall, you may be held legally at fault. You should try to prevent falls to keep your residents as healthy as possible and to avoid preventable trouble for your facility.

Should I call the doctor even if a resident falls and does not hurt himself or herself?
Yes. Those falls in which no injury occurs should be considered a warning. If we can learn from the fall and prevent future falls, the resident will be much better off. The doctor can use the circumstances of a non-injury fall to identify medication problems, physical problems, or environmental problems that can be fixed.

When should the resident who falls be transferred out of residential care?
Falls that cannot be prevented with the measures discussed above warrant a reevaluation of whether or not the resident is adequately safe in your facility. The decision to transfer is complicated, because the resident and his or her family will need to balance issues like independence and cost against the advantages of extra staffing and expertise in a nursing facility. It is best to consider the risk of falls as just one factor.

FEVER AND CHILLS

Fever is an increase in the body's normal temperature, signaling the onset of illness. Fever is often accompanied by chills.

What It Is

Under normal circumstances, the temperature of the body is held fairly steady within a very narrow range. Most of us think of a normal temperature as 98.6° F; however, everyone's "normal" may be just a bit higher or lower. A *fever* is considered present when the oral temperature is over 100° F, or 37.8° C. To generate heat, the body shivers, which we call chills.

The fever causes the skin to look flushed, with a reddish tint to the face. After the temperature starts to come down, sweat may form on the skin and scalp to help cool the person. The fever may cause a feeling of being washed out or fatigued. In residents who already have brain disease, fever may cause confusion or agitation. A high enough fever, such as above 104° F, can cause confusion, even in a resident who does not have underlying mental impairment.

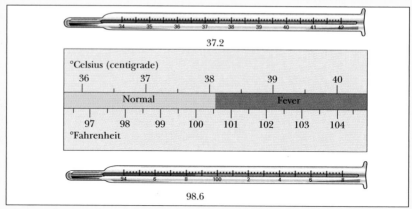

Range of normal temperature and fever.

Health Impact

Fever can be triggered by an infection, an inflammation, a cancer—in fact by many illnesses and physical problems. Often, fever is a condition that requires a doctor to do some detective work! The meaning of the fever is generally just a vague warning that something is wrong. Although under some circumstances the fever may help fight certain infections, most of the time we do not need the fever after its warning function has been served, and we then can lower the fever with medications and cool compresses. Sometimes fever results from the body's inability to effectively handle hot weather. During heat waves, many elderly persons die from *heat exhaustion* and *heatstroke*—two life-threatening reactions to being unable to adequately cool oneself. Certain drugs, discussed below, can impair a person's ability to handle hot weather and therefore increase the risk of these serious forms of illness associated with a high fever.

VARIATIONS

"Low-grade" fever of 100° to 101° F
- A feeling of being cold or chilled
- A feeling of being sick or "under the weather"
- Loss of appetite
- Sweatiness
- Fatigue

"High" fever of 102° to 106° F
- Decreased alertness
- Confusion
- Very rapid pulse or slow and weak pulse
- Seizures (a rare reaction to very high fevers)

ALERT

Any worsening of the resident's condition needs to be reported to the doctor as soon as possible. Remember: fever is just a warning sign and may reflect serious underlying problems.

MEDICATION CHECKLIST

Antipyretic Drugs. These are drugs that lower fever. Antipyretics are also pain medications, and are sometimes called analgesics. Common examples include aspirin, acetaminophen (Tylenol), and ibuprofen (Advil, many other brands).

YOUR ROLE

After the doctor is informed of the fever and the resident is evaluated, your job is to make the resident comfortable with medications, plenty of fluids, and physical care such as cool compresses. Be sure to report any change in the resident's condition to the doctor. Any change in alertness of a resident with a fever should be considered an emergency, and immediate medical attention is needed.

Hot weather can cause fever in those unable to respond normally by sweating and drinking extra fluid. Certain medications impair the body's ability to handle elevated temperature and can contribute to serious consequences such as permanent brain damage or death. Residents who take antipsychotic medication, Parkinson's disease medications, certain antidepressants, antihistamines, and drugs used for urinary incontinence are particularly likely to have an impaired ability to sweat. These residents will need extra cooling measures in very hot weather and whenever they develop a fever. Similarly, residents who take diuretics cannot conserve fluid normally to protect against dehydration, and they may require adjustment of the diuretics, extra fluids, and extra close monitoring during fevers and in hot weather.

Medical Treatment

- Examination and tests to find out what is causing the fever or chills.
- Aspirin or acetaminophen to lower temperature.
- Antibiotics to treat infection.
- The doctor may request transfer to the emergency room or hospital to allow more diagnostic tests and special care such as intravenous fluids and medications.

 DIET TIPS

- Fever causes sweating and therefore a loss of fluids—encourage the resident to drink plenty of fluids. Offer fluids every hour.
- Dietary supplements or small, frequent meals should be offered if appetite is poor.
- Alcohol use should be avoided because it can interfere with the body's ability to conserve water during a fever and therefore can contribute to dehydration.

FOR YOUR RECORDS

Health History

- Prior infections (bronchitis, bladder, etc.)
- Previous or current cancer

- Medication use
- Recent vomiting
- Recent loss of consciousness

Current Needs
- Weight monitoring
- Reporting new symptoms—cough, pain with urination, etc.—to doctor
- Adequate fluid intake
- Reporting change in alertness

COMMON QUESTIONS

How often can you give Tylenol or aspirin?
For most people, two regular strength tablets every four hours will help lower the temperature and make the person more comfortable. If you are not sure, ask the resident's doctor.

How high a temperature is "a fever"?
Most of the time, temperature under 99° F is nothing to worry about. Rectal temperature is usually almost a degree higher than oral temperature, and so we do not worry about rectal temperatures under 100° F. Temperatures are normally a bit higher in the afternoon, and also a half degree or so higher on very hot days. In general, oral temperature over 100° F and rectal temperatures over 101° F can be considered fevers.

What level of activity is appropriate for the resident with a fever?
Fever does take a toll, and in general, resting until the illness passes is a good idea. Bedrest is not necessary, however, and often being up in a chair or even sitting outside is more comfortable.

HEADACHE

The pain of a headache is a symptom that accompanies many disorders. The challenge is to decide when a headache is just a minor problem and when it signals a problem that requires a doctor's attention.

What It Is

The brain itself does not actually feel pain—a surgeon can cut into the brain without causing pain. The skull is lined with membranes, however, that are very sensitive. When these membranes and their associated blood vessels are stimulated, severe pain in the head can occur.

Headache can be caused by many things. Many headaches are due to a disease called migraine, an inherited sensitivity of the blood vessels around the brain. Although rare, headaches may be due to blood clots or even cancer in the brain. Headaches can be a side-effect of medication, or may occur after particular foods are eaten or when alcohol is consumed. Headaches also may be caused by arthritis in the neck, stress, or a head or neck injury.

Health Impact

The pain of headache can decrease the resident's pleasure in life and interfere with socialization and participation in usual activities. Associated nausea can interfere with nutrition. When a resident has a severe headache, he or she may become irritable and annoyed by any noise or contact with staff or residents. Clearly this can contribute to arguments and the potential for problems with staff and other residents.

VARIATIONS

Tension Headaches

- Most tension headaches have no warning symptoms before the headache starts.
- They are often associated with a stressful event, inadequate sleep, or a missed meal.
- These are the most common type of headache and even affect people who rarely get headaches.

Migraine Headaches

- A migraine headache is preceded by visual disturbances, called an *aura*, such as a resident seeing a bright light.
- May be accompanied by numbness or weakness of one side of the body, or by vomiting.

- Usually a family history of migraine exists, or the resident has a history of migraines in the past.
- Sensitivity to bright light and noise can be more severe during a migraine than during a common tension headache.

Withdrawal Headaches

- Caffeine withdrawal headaches are very common. Most people who drink a daily cup of coffee in the morning will get a headache if they skip coffee or other caffeinated beverages for even one day!
- Headaches can occur when a drug is stopped or is being tapered, such as an antidepressant.

Drug Side-Effect Headaches

- Many drugs can cause headache, and certain drugs like nitroglycerin tablets almost always cause a headache.

ALERT

Most often headache does not represent a brain tumor or an early sign of a stroke. There are certain characteristics of headaches, however, that suggest something serious. These include: if vomiting is present, if headaches are becoming more frequent or severe, or if the resident has developed a new problem accompanying the headache, such as difficulty in being awakened, slurring of speech, or new weakness of an arm or leg. In these cases the problem should be promptly reported to the resident's doctor. Also, any headache that is so prolonged or severe that it interferes with the resident's adequate intake of fluid or food should be reported to the doctor.

MEDICATION CHECKLIST

Analgesics (Pain Medications). For the mildest pain, acetaminophen (Tylenol, and others) or aspirin (Bayer, and others) can provide excellent relief. Another class of pain medication is the nonsteroidal anti-inflammatory drugs (NSAIDs), such as ibuprofen (Advil, Motrin,and others), naproxen (Naprosyn), indomethacin (Indocin), and others. These drugs share side-effects, which include stomach ulcers and ankle swelling. Narcotic pain medicines are occasionally used for more severe pain; narcotics include acetaminophen with codeine (Tylenol and Codeine) and hydrocodone (Vicodin). They can be constipating and can cause drowsiness and confusion.

Combination Drugs. Combinations of medications often give better relief for headaches than individual medicines. This usually means

continued on following page

continued from previous page

either aspirin or acetaminophen combined with caffeine and a sedative drug. Commonly used combination drugs include Fiorinal, Fioricet, Esgic-Plus, and Phrenilin. The side-effects of such drugs can be complicated: the caffeine can make it difficult to sleep, whereas the sedative can cause drowsiness. These are drugs that can have different effects on different individuals.

Other Drugs. Migraine headaches are treated with several special drugs not used for the more common varieties of headache. Ergot alkaloids such as Sansert, Ergostat, Cafergot and D.H.E. 45 come as tablets or suppositories and provide quick relief from a migraine. They can cause numbness, nausea, rapid or slow heartbeat, and itching. A new drug, sumatriptan (Imitrex), is used to put a quick halt to severe headaches. It is injected into the skin with its own autoinjector. It can cause flushing, fatigue, anxiety, or even chest pain as side-effects. Other drugs are used to prevent future migraines. These include the beta-blockers mentioned in the section on angina.

YOUR ROLE

Most headaches last a few hours and leave no permanent damage. If headaches are becoming more frequent or are associated with vomiting or weight loss, the doctor must be informed.

Medical Treatment
- Pain medication
- Medication to prevent headaches
- Medical testing to determine the cause of headaches, or to rule out a serious problem

Residential Care Actions
- Help resident find a quiet, dark, and comfortable environment.
- Supervise pain medication use.
- Inform doctor when headaches persist or additional symptoms, such as nausea, weakness, dizziness, or change in alertness develop with the headache.

 DIET TIPS

- Dietary supplements or small, frequent meals should be offered if appetite is poor.
- Alcohol use should be avoided.

FOR YOUR RECORDS

Health History
- Previous experience with headache
- Previous head injury
- Frequent snoring (may be a clue that breathing during sleep is impaired)
- Medication use
- Alcohol use

Current Needs
- Do headaches predictably occur if morning coffee or other caffeinated beverage is skipped? If so, your staff should be aware and make extra efforts to offer such beverages.
- Does a headache make the resident particularly irritable and potentially likely to injure another resident? If so, make every effort to provide a quiet, private place for the resident to rest during a headache.

COMMON QUESTIONS

Do certain foods trigger headaches?
Although food allergy is a very uncommon cause of headache, some people find that chocolate or mushrooms or some other food item predictably triggers a headache. Only in those situations do you need to avoid certain foods to prevent headache.

Should anything special be done for a resident who always wakes up in the morning with a bad headache?
Waking up with a headache can be a sign that breathing during sleep is interrupted. This condition, called sleep apnea, can be dangerous. A pattern of *always* waking up with a headache should be reported to the doctor.

Can headaches associated with ingestion of alcohol be prevented?
A headache after drinking alcohol, often called a hangover, can be very uncomfortable. The best method to avoid this simply involves avoiding alcohol use or dramatically cutting it down. Unfortunately, residents who abuse alcohol may find this simple solution difficult. No other remedy seems to work as well, although many have been tried.

HEART ATTACK

A heart attack (also called *myocardial infarction* or MI) is the death of muscle tissue in the heart wall, caused by a disruption of blood flow through the blood vessel or vessels that normally supply the affected muscle tissue.

Myocardial infarction (heart attack) occurs when blockage in coronary artery prevents area of heart muscle from receiving enough oxygen, and affected tissues die.

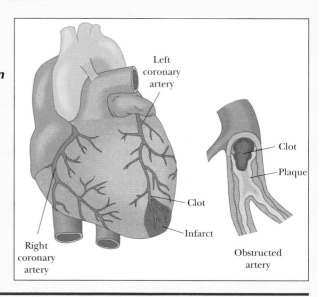

What It Is

The heart is a muscular organ that maintains the circulation of blood throughout the body by its forceful contraction or pumping action. Blood is supplied to the heart muscle by a separate network of blood vessels called the *coronary arteries*. Blockage in one or more of the coronary arteries interrupts the heart's blood supply, and the affected tissues die. The affected area, called the zone of *infarction*, no longer functions properly, and immediate treatment is required to help minimize the size of the infarction and the effect on the heart's pumping ability.

Health Impact

Approximately one half of all people who suffer a heart attack die during the first few minutes or hours. For those who survive, the risk of another heart attack is increased, although the impact on health and lifestyle will vary. For some, there may be no further problems, while for others there may be a significant weakening of the heart, fatigue, shortness of breath, episodes of chest pain, and irregularities in the heart beat.

VARIATIONS

Classic Signs and Symptoms	• Chest pain • A feeling of chest pressure or tightness • Shortness of breath • Sweating • Nausea and vomiting • A sense of impending doom or death • Pain or numbness in the jaw, left arm, or shoulder
Atypical Signs and Symptoms	• Abdominal pain • Back pain • "Silent" heart attack (this is a heart attack that causes no symptoms, or such mild or atypical symptoms that a heart attack is not suspected)
Potential Problems and Complications	• Denial of symptoms • Delayed medical attention • Sudden death

ALERT

Chest pain or pressure that is more severe or prolonged than usual, or that is not relieved by prescribed medication, such as nitroglycerin, needs to be reported to the doctor or your local emergency medical services (EMS) system immediately.

MEDICATION CHECKLIST

Nitrates. Nitrates are used to increase blood flow to the heart. They can be used under the tongue (to work extra fast), as a skin patch, as a spray, and as pills. Common examples include nitroglycerin (which comes as tablets, a spray, skin patches, and ointments) and isosorbide dinitrate (Isordil).

Vasodilators. These drugs expand the blood vessels, letting blood flow more easily and reducing the heart's work. They also may reduce chest pain and lower the risk of a future heart attack. Examples are the ACE inhibitors, calcium channel blockers, beta blockers, and hydralazine. Common ACE inhibitors are enalapril (Vasotec), lisinopril (Prinivil, Zestril), and others. A related medicine is losartan

continued on following page

> *continued from previous page*
> (Cozaar). Common calcium channel blocking drugs are nifedipine (Adalat CC, Procardia XL), diltiazem (Cardizem), verapamil (Calan, Isoptin), and many others. Common beta blockers are propranolol (Inderal), metoprolol (Lopressor, Toprol), atenolol (Tenormin), and others.

YOUR ROLE

Your role for a resident who is having a heart attack is to get medical help immediately. This usually involves calling 911, but some residents who have other medical conditions such as dementia or cancer may have advance directives against hospitalization. In such cases, the doctor will have to instruct you in advance (if you have no instructions you should call for help immediately). Sometimes the symptoms of a heart attack are subtle or confusing. If you have any doubt, contact the doctor for guidance.

After Hospitalization

After a resident recovers from a heart attack, a program of heart rehabilitation is begun. This may require trips back to the hospital or another care facility for supervised exercise and testing, as well as specific activities that must be performed in your facility. It is important to remember that these residents have had a life-threatening experience, and some emotional adjustment, as well as lifestyle changes, will be required. For example, it is not uncommon for some level of depression to be experienced. You can serve an important role in supporting a resident's adjustments during this period and by notifying the doctor if the resident seems depressed.

Medical Treatment

- Hospitalization
- Oxygen
- Bedrest
- Medications
- Surgery in selected cases

Residential Care Actions

- Weight monitoring.
- Limit alcohol use.
- Supervise medications.
- Gradually increase activity, as prescribed by the doctor.

DIET TIPS

- Low-sodium (salt) diet is often prescribed by doctor.
- Extra potassium in diet *only if prescribed.*
- Extra fiber and fluids if constipation present.
- Dietary supplements or small, frequent meals can be offered if appetite is poor.
- Alcohol use should be discussed with the doctor. Often one or two drinks per day are permitted, but there may be a problem with one of the medications. If in doubt, ask the doctor!

FOR YOUR RECORDS

Health History
- Previous heart attacks
- High blood pressure
- Medication use
- Alcohol use
- Weight
- Height
- Chest pain
- Shortness of breath

Current Needs
- Monitor freshness of nitroglycerin—it must not be outdated or improperly stored.
- Monitor weight.
- Keep list of doctors, ambulance, and hospital preferences current.
- Support efforts to stop smoking, lose weight, and exercise.

COMMON QUESTIONS

How long can someone live after having a heart attack?
Although about one fourth of people who have a heart attack die before they get to the hospital, most people who have a heart attack get better and return home. They do have a higher risk than average of having another heart attack, but medical treatment and lifestyle changes can improve that. In fact, some people live many years after a heart attack, and so it is important to have a positive attitude about doing well.

Does a person always have chest pain with a heart attack?
No. Some people have absolutely no symptoms at all. Other symptoms may include feeling "under the weather," nausea, or pain in the arm or jaw without chest pain. Any change in a resident's condition that makes you wonder if something serious is going on should be reported to the doctor.

What level of activity is appropriate after a heart attack?
Immediately during and after a heart attack, the resident will need to rest in bed. This usually is done in the hospital, but sometimes the doctor will decide that staying at home is in the resident's best interest, and you will be advised regarding proper activity. After the heart muscle has started to heal, activity is gradually increased until the resident's activity level is back to or as close to normal as possible. The rate of increase will be determined by the doctor. Sometimes the doctor will prescribe a special exercise.

What should I do when I think someone is having a heart attack?
Call for emergency services, usually by dialing 911.

HIGH BLOOD PRESSURE

High blood pressure, or hypertension, is a sustained increase in the amount of pressure required to keep blood moving through the circulation.

What It Is

The heart is a pump whose job is to pump blood to the muscles, brain, kidneys, and other internal organs. The blood must be ejected from the heart with enough pressure to reach all of these organs, and the pressure is normally controlled by tiny muscles in the walls of the blood vessels that squeeze or relax as needed to ensure the correct flow of blood. For reasons that are unknown, some people develop too much squeezing of these muscles, leading to too much pressure inside the blood vessels. It is likely that in many cases the tendency to have high blood pressure is inherited, but additional factors that contribute to high blood pressure are smoking, drinking too much alcohol, being overweight, and not getting enough exercise.

Health Impact

If you lift heavy weights every day, soon the muscles in your arms will become thick and enlarged. The heart is a muscle, and the "weight" it lifts is blood. If the blood pressure is higher than normal over a period of years, the heart muscle becomes thickened and the heart enlarges. This thickening reduces the pumping ability of the heart (see Congestive Heart Failure) and increases the risk of a heart attack. High blood pressure damages the tiny blood vessels in the brain and kidneys, and causes fatty deposits to accumulate in large blood vessels, contributing to heart attacks, strokes, and kidney failure.

High blood pressure is called a "silent" disease, meaning that usually there are no symptoms to warn of danger until serious damage has been done. Only by early identification and treatment of high blood pressure can serious health problems be prevented.

VARIATIONS

Early Symptoms

There are no early symptoms of high blood pressure. This is why it is sometimes called "the silent killer."

Advanced Symptoms

- Dizziness
- Ankle swelling
- Shortness of breath with exercise
- Headache
- Sleepiness
- Blurred vision
- Confusion

Potential Problems and Complications

- Stroke
- Heart attack
- Kidney failure

ALERT

Sometimes medication can lower blood pressure too much, especially if the resident has had a poor fluid intake or fluid loss from vomiting or diarrhea. The doctor must be informed of any symptoms of dizziness or light-headedness or any fainting.

MEDICATION CHECKLIST

Diuretics. Commonly called water pills, diuretics actually help get rid of excess salt *and* water. They can limit swelling of the legs and the collection of salty water in the lungs. Common examples include hydrochlorothiazide, and triamterene/hydrochlorothiazide (Dyazide).

Beta Blockers. These medications slow the heart and reduce the force of pumping actions. Common examples include atenolol (Tenormin) and metoprolol (Lopressor).

Vasodilators. These medications expand the blood vessels, letting blood flow more easily and easing the heart's work. Examples are the ACE inhibitors, calcium channel blockers, losartan, and hydralazine. The ACE inhibitors, including enalopril (Vasotec), captopril (Capoten), lisinopril (Zestril, Prinovil), and many others, can cause a long-lasting cough, rash, or swelling of the lips or face. The calcium channel blockers, including nifedepine (Procardia, Adalat), diltiazem (Cardizem), verapamil (Calan, Isoptin), and others, can cause swelling of the ankles or constipation. All of these drugs can cause light-headedness or dizziness.

continued on next page

continued from previous page

Alpha Blockers. These drugs block nerve impulses that tighten blood vessels. Common examples include prazocin (Minipress), doxazosin (Cardura), and terazocin (Hytrin). They can cause light-headedness or dizziness.

Centrally Active Drugs. These drugs work in a variety of ways to lower blood pressure. They can be pills such as methyldopa (Aldomet), guanfacine (Tenex), or clondine (Catapres), or can be a skin patch (Catapres-TTS).

YOUR ROLE

Because a resident does not "feel" high blood pressure, he or she may forget or refuse to take medication. Encouragement is important to help residents comply with treatment.

Medical Treatment
- Diet and lifestyle counseling
- Exercise
- High blood pressure medications

 DIET TIPS

- Low-sodium (salt) diet generally prescribed by doctor
- Extra potassium in diet *only if prescribed*

FOR YOUR RECORDS

Health History
- Previous stroke, heart attack, or kidney failure
- Previous high blood pressure
- Medication use
- Alcohol use
- Recent blood pressure values

Current Needs
- Weight monitoring.
- Support efforts to stop smoking.
- Limit alcohol use.
- Encourage regular medication use.
- Report any evidence of medication side-effects.

COMMON QUESTIONS

If high blood pressure does not cause any symptoms, why take medication that may be expensive or cause side-effects?
There is excellent evidence that treating high blood pressure can prevent strokes, heart failure, and premature death. The long-term benefits are so significant that it is worth the expense and trouble of taking a medication.

With so many choices, how does the doctor choose a high blood pressure medication?
Each family of high blood pressure medication has its own side-effects. Some medications are more likely to work for a particular age group or racial group. Cost and convenience are also important factors. Often, when one medication fails to control high blood pressure, the doctor may add a second medication. Sometimes a combination of medicines works better.

What level of activity is appropriate for the resident with high blood pressure?
Physical activity can help lower blood pressure, and exercise should be encouraged. Some individuals with high blood pressure have light-headedness when they stand up. Such residents should be encouraged to rise slowly and to dangle their legs over the side of the bed before getting up.

KIDNEY FAILURE

Kidney failure is the inability of the kidneys to filter the body's blood and rid the body of toxic waste products.

What It Is

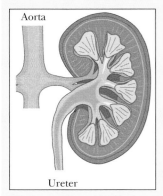

Aorta

Ureter

Cross-section of kidney, which filters waste products from the blood.

The body's blood supply carries important nutrients and other substances throughout the body and removes waste products. Normally, the kidneys filter the blood continuously to remove waste products.

Disease or injury can reduce the kidneys'capacity for filtration, thereby causing fluids, waste products, and other substances to build up in the body. Problems damaging the kidneys that cannot be cured, including diabetes, uncontrolled high blood pressure, effects of some medications, or severe injury can cause kidney failure.

At present there are only two forms of treatment for kidney failure—kidney transplant and dialysis.

Health Impact

When the kidneys fail, salty water builds up in the ankles, lower legs, and in some cases the lungs and bowels. This buildup of salt can cause high blood pressure, and the accumulated waste products lead to lack of energy, poor appetite, and easy tiring. The waste products also cause impaired sleep and daytime sleepiness. Drugs that are normally eliminated by the kidney can build up, causing dangerous side-effects. Also the body does not heal well, and infections are harder for the body to resist.

This means that attention must be paid to everything going into the body and everything coming out. As the damaged kidneys have trouble handling extra salt or potassium, often special diets are needed to spare the damaged kidney the chore of eliminating the excess. Because the waste products of protein cannot be eliminated, the doctor may also limit the protein content of the diet.

Dialysis

Kidney dialysis requires access to the blood several times a week, and this repeated access is accomplished by the surgical placement of a shunt that makes getting into the blood vessels easier.

A blocked shunt, which may be caused by blood clots, is an emergency and requires an immediate call to the doctor.

Peritoneal dialysis is an alternative that allows many people with kidney failure to be dialyzed at home. It involves the placement of sterile salt water into the abdominal cavity through a tube, and then draining the water after waste products have had a chance to flow into it. If an infection develops from this procedure, the resident can get very sick; therefore, any fever or change in the resident's condition is cause for concern and requires medical attention.

VARIATIONS

Early Symptoms
- Ankle swelling
- Shortness of breath with exercise
- Fatigue
- Weakness
- Increased urination at night

Advanced Symptoms

These would usually be present only in someone with kidney disease advanced enough to be under the care of a doctor.

- Weight gain due to fluid accumulation
- Swelling of the lower legs and feet
- Loss of appetite
- Puffy face or eyelids
- Inability to sleep well or excessive sleepiness
- Confusion

Potential Problems and Complications
- Poor healing of minor cuts or infections
- Coma
- Death

ALERT

Weighing the resident frequently can provide important clues that extra salt is being retained. Ask the doctor how much weight change should be reported.

MEDICATION CHECKLIST

Diuretics. Commonly called water pills, diuretics actually help get rid of excess salt *and* water. They can limit the swelling of the legs and the collection of salty water in the lungs. Common examples used in kidney failure include furosemide (Lasix) and bumetanide (Bumex).

Aluminum Antacids. This medicine binds to and helps eliminate one of the waste products that builds up in kidney failure.

Anti-Rejection Drugs. These medicines fight the normal tendency of the body to reject a transplanted organ. They also can impair the body's ability to fight infection. Common examples include cyclosporine and prednisone.

YOUR ROLE

There is no perfect substitute for well-functioning kidneys. Even transplanting a new kidney into the body of a person with kidney failure requires a lifetime of medications to prevent the body from rejecting it, as well as careful monitoring of kidney function on a regular basis. In kidney failure, doctors attempt to manage what goes into and out of the body to substitute for the natural, normal function of the kidneys. Controlling diet is important. Extra salt in the diet can lead to weight gain, increased swelling of the legs or ankles, or shortness of breath. Help make sure that the resident does not cheat on the diet by eating salty snacks. The diet is likely also to be limited in potassium and protein. This may require consulting a registered dietitian. The resident's kidney specialist may be able to help with this, and many dialysis units also employ a dietitian who can be helpful.

The resident with kidney failure will have less ability to fight infections, and illness can become serious very rapidly. A change in alertness, fever, or other change in condition warrants a call to the doctor.

Medical Treatment

- Special diet: restricted sodium (salt), potassium, and protein
- Medication to help eliminate certain waste products
- Dose adjustment of other medications to compensate for reduced clearance by the kidneys
- Dialysis to artificially filter the kidneys
- Transplantation to provide a new kidney surgically

Residential Care Actions

- Weight monitoring
- For resident on dialysis: coordinating transportation to dialysis facility and communication with dialysis staff
- Prompt contact with the doctor regarding any infection or other change in resident's condition

 DIET TIPS

- A low sodium (salt), potassium, and protein diet is generally prescribed by doctor.
- Provide extra fiber if constipation present.
- Provide dietary supplements or extra portions of food if appetite is poor.
- Alcohol use should be avoided.

FOR YOUR RECORDS

Health History

- Heart attack
- High blood pressure
- Medication use
- Alcohol use

Current Needs

- Extra pillows for sleep
- Sleep aids and night light
- Hygiene aids for urinary incontinence

COMMON QUESTIONS

How long can someone live with kidney failure?
Although kidney failure can and does kill, when treated successfully people can live for many years. If treated with dialysis or kidney transplant, the person with kidney failure can live a normal life span.

Why does the doctor not give enough of the diuretics (water pills) to produce enough urine to completely get rid of the waste products?
The water pills have their own side-effects, and using too much of them can actually worsen kidney failure or cause painful arthritis (called gout). Using too much of the water pills can also result in light-headedness and fainting spells.

MOVEMENT DISORDERS AND SEIZURES

Diseases of the brain can result in difficulty with movement, causing normally simple activities like walking or brushing the teeth to become significant challenges. Some of these movement disorders cause uncontrollable shaking of the limbs, called *tremors.* Some brain diseases can result in a massive electrical discharge in the brain, with uncontrollable movements and even loss of consciousness. This abnormal electrical activity of the brain is called a *seizure.*

An important difference between seizures and movement disorders is that movement disorders affect residents all the time. A resident with a seizure disorder will behave and move entirely normally when not having a seizure.

What It Is

The control of movement by the brain is very complicated, and there are many diseases in which this control is damaged or altered. The following disorders produce movement problems that are present most of the time and are therefore considered *chronic.* The most common disorder seen in residential care is Parkinson's disease, in which there is a slowing of movement, shaking of the limbs, and a significantly increased risk of falls. Another common movement disorder is called *essential tremor,* in which the resident shakes when a limb is being actively used. Some residents will have slow, writhing movements of their face or tongue, due to a condition called *tardive dyskinesia.* This movement disorder can occur for unknown reasons, but often it occurs as a side-effect of medications such as antipsychotic drugs.

Seizure disorders occur when sudden, massive electrical discharges in the brain result in shaking of all the limbs and loss of consciousness. Other forms of seizures can look different, but the underlying electrical process in the brain is similar. The other forms of seizure may cause a resident to experience a brief loss of awareness or movement, or to have a brief and uncontrollable movement of a limited area of the body, such as "smacking" of the lips.

Health Impact

As there are many movement disorders, there are many different degrees and patterns of impairment. Parkinson's disease causes a general slowness of movement. Balance is impaired, and posture tends to be stooped. Walking is impaired, with small steps required to maintain balance. In addition, the resident may develop constipation, skin rashes, loss of memory, and an increased sensitivity to medicines that affect the brain.

Essential tremor can produce very noticeable shaking whenever a resident uses the arms and hands, but it rarely causes much difficulty in accomplishing activities of daily living (although it can result in problems holding a cup of liquid without spilling). Essential tremor does not progressively get worse in the way Parkinson's disease does.

Tardive dyskinesia can interfere with eating and thus result in malnutrition. It can produce social isolation, as other residents may avoid the resident because of his or her "strange" movements.

A person with a seizure disorder generally shows no evidence of the problem between seizures. When a seizure occurs, the resident can fall and is at risk for injuries (cuts, bruises, broken bones). Some people lose bladder control during a seizure, and after a seizure, it is common for the individual to have a period of sleepiness or weakness of part of the body. This is called the *post-ictal state*.

VARIATIONS

Signs and Symptoms	• Slowness or awkward-appearing movement • Stooped posture • Uncontrollable shaking of the arms and legs • Uncontrollable protruding of the tongue
Movement Disorders	• Shaking (tremor) in Parkinson's disease and essential tremor • Slowness of movement in Parkinson's disease • Rigidity in Parkinson's disease • Difficulty drinking liquids without spilling in essential tremor • Facial movements interfering with eating in tardive dyskinesia
Seizures	• Generally occur in an unpredictable fashion
Parkinson's Disease	• Dementia • Dry, flaky skin on the forehead • Constipation • Stooped posture • Poor balance • Trouble handling saliva, tendency to drool
Potential Problems and Complications	• Inability to do self-care activities

ALERT

A seizure that lasts unusually long or is different from the resident's "usual" seizure in some way should be brought to the doctor's attention. In residents who are known to have a seizure disorder, it is rarely necessary to call 911 unless an injury occurs during a seizure. Understand that between seizures a resident should have normal movements unless another disease state is present. New falling or difficulty walking may reflect a side-effect of the seizure medication and should be called to the attention of the doctor.

MEDICATION CHECKLIST

Antiparkinson Drugs. These help with the shaking and slow movements of Parkinson's disease. Common examples include levodopa (Sinemet), bromocriptine (Parlodel), and pergolide (Permax).

Anticonvulsant Drugs. These medications help prevent seizures. Common examples include phenytoin (Dilantin), carbamazepine (Tegretol), and phenobarbital.

YOUR ROLE

Caring for residents with movement disorders or seizures means making your facility as physically safe as possible. Extra care needs to be taken to ensure that sharp edges of furniture are cushioned, and that edges of rugs and exposed electrical cords are eliminated to help prevent falls. Handrails and elevated toilet seats may help safe movement and toileting. If a movement disorder makes a resident slow in walking or getting out of a chair, he or she will need extra attention in case of fire or earthquake or any situation requiring immediate evacuation. Your staff will need to be trained to handle such individuals in case of emergency.

For residents with a seizure disorder, ask the doctor in advance what measures should be taken when a seizure occurs. Reassure the other residents, because there might be a fear of seizures and "odd" movements that might cause these residents to be isolated. For residents with other movement disorders, inform your staff about any extra help the resident might need for routine self-care.

Medical Treatment

- Medication to prevent seizures or help manage movement disorders
- Physical therapy as indicated

 DIET TIPS

- Swallowing can be impaired in certain movement disorders. If coughing while eating develops, inform the doctor.
- Dietary supplements or small, frequent meals should be offered if appetite is poor.
- Food can alter the absorption of medications used to treat Parkinson's disease. Ask the doctor when the medicine should be given.
- Alcohol use should be minimized. Alcohol can reduce the shaking of essential tremor temporarily, and unfortunately, this can lead to excess alcohol use in some individuals.

FOR YOUR RECORDS

Health History

- Previous seizures
- Prior stroke (which can complicate movement disorders and increase risk of seizures)
- Dementia
- Nature and severity of symptoms; frequency of seizures
- Self-care abilities and needs
- Urinary incontinence
- Medication use
- Alcohol use

Current Needs

- Weight monitoring
- Safety precautions
- Medication supervision

COMMON QUESTIONS

My other residents become frightened when one of the residents has a seizure. How can I help?

Although the frequency of seizures can be minimized with medications, they often cannot be completely prevented. It is necessary to reassure the other residents and, if possible, teach them the nature of the problem. This helps prevent unfair treatment by the other residents. It may help to instruct other residents about what to do if the resident does have a seizure. They need to know whom to call, and specific actions to take such as whether or not a tongue protector is needed to prevent the resident from biting the tongue.

A resident with Parkinson's disease seems to be getting steadily worse. Isn't the medication working anymore?
There currently is no treatment for Parkinson's disease that prevents progression of the disease. All the medications tend to help initially with the movement disorder, but lose their effect as time goes on. In general, side-effects of the medicines become more of a problem with time, and the benefit of the treatment decreases. Because it is a progressive disease, you need to periodically reevaluate whether your facility can adequately provide for the resident's needs.

What level of activity is safe for the resident with a movement disorder?
Staying active is an important goal for anyone with Parkinson's disease and other movement disorders. Residents should be encouraged to remain as physically active as possible. To that end, your facility should be made safe and helpful for such residents.

MUSCLE OR BONE PAIN

Aches and pains in the muscles, arms, legs, back, and neck are very common, and most of us are comfortable treating them with medications that can be bought without prescription, such as aspirin, or by applying heat or cold to the painful area. However, you may have to help a resident and contact the doctor when an ache or pain does not respond to these common measures.

What It Is

Pain is a warning the body uses to let us know an injury or illness is present. It can help protect us by calling attention to the problem so appropriate protective measures can be taken or the necessary medical care can be obtained.

Unfortunately, some conditions are associated with pain that persists or interferes with daily life. Arthritis, low back pain, and certain broken bones in the spine (called *compression fractures*) are usually treated by using measures to limit the pain.

Health Impact

Pain impairs the resident's ability to enjoy life and participate in usual activities. Pain can cause loss of appetite and interfere with nutrition. If self-care is limited by pain, hygiene can suffer and the resident may develop skin problems and body odor. Pain can lead to depression as well.

VARIATIONS

Moderate Pain
- Aching muscles
- Pain after exercising or walking an extra long distance
- Pain after a minor fall or injury
- Symptoms that usually respond to over-the-counter medication

Severe Pain
- Pain that cannot be easily explained, that lasts longer or is more severe than usual
- Pain that interferes with a resident's sleep or appetite
- Pain that leads to depression

Problems Requiring Immediate Medical Attention
- Sudden severe pain
- Pain that interferes with bearing weight (standing, walking)
- Pain that prevents the resident from getting out of bed
- Pain associated with nausea, vomiting, or a change in alertness

ALERT

Black or tarry bowel movements or vomiting blood in any resident is an emergency. This can occur when certain pain medications in the aspirin family cause stomach or intestinal ulcers.

MEDICATION CHECKLIST

Analgesics (Pain Medications). For the mildest pain, acetaminophen (Tylenol, and others) or aspirin (Bayer, and others) can provide excellent relief. Another class of pain medications are the non-steroidal anti-inflammatory drugs (NSAIDs), such as ibuprofen (Advil, Motrin, and others), naproxen (Naprosyn), indomethacin (Indocin), and others. These drugs share side-effects, which include stomach ulcers and ankle swelling. Narcotic pain medicines are occasionally used for more severe pain; narcotics include acetaminophen with codeine (Tylenol and Codeine) and hydrocodone (Vicodin). They can be constipating and can cause drowsiness and confusion.

YOUR ROLE

First decide if the pain requires immediate attention. If not, inform the doctor as soon as possible if the pain is anything more than the most minor injury. Have medication for routine and minor pains, such as aspirin, acetaminophen, or ibuprofen. If a resident is prescribed a narcotic medication, be aware that severe constipation may develop, and help the resident drink extra fluids and eat more fiber.

When a resident has pain that does not get better as fast as you expect, contact the doctor. Any injury that interferes with the resident's function (ability to walk, dress, feed himself or herself) should always be considered important enough to contact the doctor. Inform the doctor any time a resident seems to be getting sleepy, dizzy, or confused from pain medication.

Medical Treatment
- Diagnostic tests to determine the cause of the pain
- Pain medication
- Heating pads, cold packs

DIET TIPS

- Extra fiber and fluid if constipation present and especially if codeine or other narcotics are being used.
- Dietary supplements or small, frequent meals if appetite is poor.
- Alcohol use should be avoided.

FOR YOUR RECORDS

Health History
- Previous falls
- Easy bruising
- Medication use; pain medication use, especially excess use
- Alcohol use

Current Needs
- Weight monitoring
- Monitoring functional status

COMMON QUESTIONS

What is the difference between aspirin and Tylenol?
For most purposes, they are about the same. When swelling is present, as after an ankle is sprained, aspirin has more of an anti-inflammatory effect and will help reduce the swelling. However, aspirin also causes more stomach problems than Tylenol and is best avoided if ulcer disease is present. If in doubt, ask the doctor for a recommendation.

Which is better after an injury—ice or heat?
Ice helps reduce the swelling that occurs immediately after an injury, such as twisting or spraining an ankle. After the initial injury, heat can improve blood flow to the injured area and helps relax tight muscles. A heating pad can feel wonderful when a back is injured, for example. However, great care needs to be taken with heating pads for elderly or mentally impaired residents and for any resident with damage to the nerves from diabetes or a stroke, because these individuals can easily be burned. Heating pad use should be closely supervised. Put the heating pad on top of the affected area, instead of placing the resident's

weight on the heating pad. Be sure to put the heating pad in a protective cover.

The pain is much better, but a large bruise has developed below the area of injury. What should I do?
It may take several days for the blood that forms a bruise to work its way toward the skin, where it can be seen. Often by this time the pain is reduced, and the new bruise worries staff. One clue is that as bruises start to heal they change color, first purple, then brown, then even a greenish tint can be seen before the bruise disappears. If the pain is getting better, a bruise with brown or green coloring that is found a few days later under the area of injury is not cause for additional worry.

NAUSEA AND VOMITING

Vomiting is a reflex controlled by a vomiting center in the brain. It is an uncontrollable muscular action that causes the stomach contents to be forcefully expelled. Nausea, an uncomfortable feeling in the stomach area, usually occurs before vomiting. Nausea, however, can occur without ever becoming strong enough to produce vomiting.

What It Is

Nausea and vomiting can be a protective response to poisoning, letting the body eliminate dangerous substances, such as poisons and spoiled food. Vomiting also can be a response to many forms of illness. Unfortunately, many other situations trigger nausea.

Nausea is a side-effect of many medications, including heart pills, antibiotics, and iron pills.

Nausea and vomiting can occur when the bowel or stomach is blocked by constipation or bowel disease. A common problem may occur years after adominal surgery if loops of bowel get caught in scar tissue, called *adhesions*, causing bowel blockage and severe nausea.

Pneumonia, viruses, infections of the stomach, ulcers, brain tumors, strokes, and other illnesses can cause nausea and vomiting. Nausea is a problem that requires further investigation, usually by the doctor.

Health Impact

Besides being uncomfortable, nausea can lead to poor nutrition and even depression if it is long-lasting. Vomiting can cause the body to lose important salts, thereby disturbing the body's normal chemical and fluid balance and producing symptoms such as weakness and confusion. If enough vomiting occurs, dehydration can develop. This can lead to fainting, weakness, and, if severe enough, kidney failure. Nausea and vomiting can affect the resident's ability to ingest or absorb medications. Prolonged nausea and vomiting can lead to inadequate food intake and poor nutrition.

Two complications of vomiting are particularly dangerous. If vomit accidently enters the windpipe and therefore gains access to the lungs, the acid in the vomit can seriously burn the delicate lung tissue. This is called *aspiration* and can result in a particularly serious form of pneumonia. The risk of aspiration can be reduced by helping position the resident's head while vomiting to minimize the chance of vomit entering the windpipe. The second complication of vomiting occurs when persistent vomiting disturbs the chemical balance of the body. This can initially leave the resident mentally confused and weak and, if uncorrected, can be fatal. Hospitalization and intravenous fluid might be needed to restore chemical balance to the body.

VARIATIONS

Symptoms
- A queasy feeling
- Loss of appetite
- Gagging

Potential Problems and Complications
- Aspirating (inhaling) vomit into windpipe or lungs
- Dehydration
- Malnutrition
- Kidney failure

ALERT

Vomiting blood is a medical emergency and needs to be reported to the doctor immediately. Unless you have prior instructions from the doctor, call an ambulance or 911.

MEDICATION CHECKLIST

Antiemetic Drugs. These drugs help calm the centers in the brain that control the feeling of nausea. They are usually used only when the underlying cause of the nausea cannot be eliminated. Common examples include trimethobenzamide (Tigan) and prochlorperazine (Compazine). These drugs can be given in pill form or as a suppository.

YOUR ROLE

A resident who suddenly develops nausea and vomiting needs medical attention, and your role is to see that this occurs without delay to avoid dehydration or chemical imbalances. Remind the doctor of medications the resident is taking, because vomiting could be an important side-effect. (This is easier if you prepare a list before calling the doctor.) If several residents develop nausea and vomiting, make sure that your staff follows proper food handling and storage techniques.

Some residents have long-standing nausea. These residents will need your help to ensure adequate nutrition. You will need to determine when a change occurs in their usual status, and make sure they get medical attention when such a change occurs. You may be asked to help give medication to control the nausea when symptoms are particularly severe.

Medical Treatment

- Identifying the cause of nausea and vomiting
- Medications or other treatment to eliminate the cause of the nausea and vomiting
- Pills, shots, or suppositories to decrease the nausea
- Replacement fluids and/or salts either by mouth or through an intravenous line

 DIET TIPS

- Bland foods
- Replacement fluids
- Extra potassium or sodium in diet *only if prescribed*
- Extra fiber if constipation present
- Dietary supplements or small, frequent meals if appetite is poor
- Alcohol use should be avoided

FOR YOUR RECORDS

Health History

- Previous abdominal surgery, cancer or chemotherapy, head injury, or vomiting
- Medications
- Alcohol use

Current Needs

- Weight monitoring
- Monitoring bowel movements and urination patterns
- Maintaining dietary intake

COMMON QUESTIONS

When should the doctor be informed that a resident is nauseated?
Contact the doctor whenever a resident vomits, and whenever nausea without vomiting interferes with the resident drinking enough fluids or eating enough food. If several residents develop vomiting, consider the possibility that food poisoning is occurring, and contact your local public health officer to help identify and prevent future problems.

What types of food are good to offer a nauseated resident?
Dry toast, plain rice, and baked potatoes are examples of bland food that are easy to digest. Often foods that are spicy or have strong odors are particularly hard for a nauseated person to hold down. Cool water, flat ginger ale, or sugared sport drinks are fluids that can be offered. Note that the sugar content of these drinks may not be appropriate for diabetic residents.

POOR SLEEP

Sleep problems may take the form of an inability to fall asleep quickly, to stay asleep through the night, or having nightmares that disrupt sleep frequently.

What It Is

Some sleep problems are simply a result of poor sleep habits. Residents learn to fear going to sleep, because they have had difficulty in the past. They become more and more anxious about sleep, and end up with impaired sleep patterns. Other residents truly have a disease process that affects sleep. This can be a side-effect of a medication or the presence of certain sleep diseases such as "restless legs" or sleep apnea. When sleep is impaired, the doctor must be notified for an evaluation of the cause of the sleep problem.

Sleep habits differ between people, and a wide variety of sleep patterns can be considered normal. Whereas for one person it might be normal to fall asleep at 7 P.M. and sleep to 6 A.M., it may be equally normal for someone else to take a short afternoon nap, then fall asleep at midnight and sleep until 9 A.M. The quality and quantity of our sleep change as we age, and satisfaction with sleep decreases as we get older. The important fact to remember is that a change in sleep patterns should be considered abnormal and worth investigating. Often the change can be linked to a new medicine, to depression, or to other treatable conditions.

Health Impact

Sleep is an altered level of mental function that generally is needed to refresh the mind and body. Very important brain activities occur during sleep and, if enough sleep is missed, daytime functioning can be severely impaired.

Poor sleep can cause daytime sleepiness, fatigue, and confusion. Poor sleep can be a sign of depression, but poor sleep can also lead to depression. The sleep-deprived resident will be sleepier during the day and is more likely to be sensitive to the sedating side-effects of drugs. This can contribute to an increased risk of falls and accidents. Certain problems with sleep can contribute to serious heart problems and even death.

VARIATIONS

Signs and Symptoms

- Difficulty falling asleep
- Waking up early and being unable to fall back to sleep

- Waking up frequently during the night
- Never feeling well rested
- Being excessively sleepy during the day

Occasional Sleep Problems

- Occasional difficulty falling asleep
- Waking up several times a night, but having no trouble getting back to sleep

Persistent Sleep Problems

- Difficulty falling asleep almost every night
- Staying awake much of the night
- Waking up early in the morning and being unable to fall back asleep
- Feeling tired all day
- Shifting of sleep so that the hours that the resident sleeps do not correspond to when the other residents sleep

Potential Problems and Complications

- Poor quality of life due to severe fatigue and discomfort from poor sleep
- Mental confusion from inadequate sleep

ALERT

Sudden development of severe sleepiness during the day should be reported to the doctor immediately.

MEDICATION CHECKLIST

Sleeping Pills. Sleeping pills can help the resident go to sleep faster or stay asleep better. Unfortunately, the benefit diminishes after a few weeks of regular use, and they are best used for short periods of time or only occasionally rather than every night. Medications also have side-effects, such as daytime sleepiness and increased risk of confusion and falls. If used every night, there may be withdrawal effects when the medication is stopped. These withdrawal effects can include worsening of the sleep problem that prompted their use. Common examples of sleeping pills include triazolam (Halcion), temazepam (Restoril), and zolpidem (Ambien). Several antihistamines are available without a prescription for use as sleeping pills. These over-the-counter drugs can have side-effects that make them particularly poor choices for elderly residents—dry mouth, constipation, difficulty urinating, and confusion. Examples include doxylamine succinate (Unisom), diphenhydramine (Sominex, Nytol, Compoz), and others.

Levodopa. This medication, usually administered as a combination of levodopa and carbidopa (Sinemet, Sinemet CR), can improve abnormal leg movements and discomfort that can impair sleep.

YOUR ROLE

Some problems with sleep require a doctor's evaluation. In particular, excessive sleepiness during the day should be evaluated. It may be due to a drug side-effect, but could also represent a serious medical problem. Difficulty falling or staying asleep should be considered a possible sign of depression and should be reported to the doctor. Mild problems with sleep may represent a failure of good sleep habits, and you can help by offering residents interesting activities during the day and early evening to help them stay up until a normal bedtime after 9 or 10 P.M. At that time, they will need quiet and dark bedrooms to minimize distractions. Evening alcohol use should be discouraged among residents with sleep problems.

If an "as needed" sleeping pill is prescribed, the use of the medication should be supervised. If the resident insists on using it every night, let the doctor know because this may not be the doctor's intention.

Medical Treatment
- Counseling on better sleep habits
- Medication to aid sleep
- Medications to treat restless legs or jerky leg movements that interfere with sleep
- Pain medication to treat pain that interferes with sleep
- Changing medication that interferes with sleep

 DIET TIPS

- Fluid restriction after dinner only if approved by the doctor.
- Avoiding heavy evening meals or large late night snacks if sleep is a problem.
- Alcohol use should be avoided.

FOR YOUR RECORDS

Health History
- Previous sleep problems, depression, prostate problems, need to urinate frequently at night, snoring
- Medication use
- Alcohol use

Current Needs
- Activities to help keep residents up and occupied in the afternoon and after dinner
- Encouraging residents to avoid alcohol in the evening
- Keeping facility dark and quiet at night
- Encouraging residents to wake up at the same time every day
- Encouraging physical activity and exercise during the day
- Supervised use of sleeping pills

COMMON QUESTIONS

How much sleep does a person need?
Although the amount of sleep needed differs for everyone, the amount of sleep needed generally is eight to nine hours per night. To measure the adequacy of sleep, doctors look at how sleepy a person is during the day. If a resident is never sleepy during the day, and never naps, then sleep is sufficient no matter how much time is spent asleep.

Should fluids be restricted in the evening to prevent the resident from needing to go to the bathroom at night?
Evening fluid restriction might sometimes be prescribed by the doctor to help limit the need for nighttime urination. The total amount of fluid the resident drinks during the day, however, is quite limited, and the resident could become dehydrated. Only limit fluids in residents for whom the doctor agrees that dehydration is not a problem.

When is a sleeping pill needed?
Sleeping pills are best used for temporary or occasional problems with sleep. They rarely work well when taken on a daily basis, and they are associated with many possible side-effects.

Is a nightcap good for sleep?
Alcohol causes drowsiness and can make falling asleep easier. It causes abnormal sleep, however, with impairment in the normal function of sleep to fully refresh. A common problem when taking alcohol at night is to wake up in the middle of the night and be unable to go back to sleep. A dangerous solution to that problem would be to drink more alcohol to get back to sleep, which can easily lead to alcohol abuse. It is best to avoid evening alcohol use if sleep is at all a problem.

PRESSURE ULCERS

Healing pressure ulcer

A pressure ulcer is damaged skin in an area where the body weight is supported over a hard, bony area. Pressure ulcers can range from small reddened areas to deep craters. They often occur over the hips, buttocks, tailbone, heels, ankles, and shoulder blades. They account for more than $5 billion a year in health care expenditures, and more than 17,000 lawsuits. When a resident develops a pressure ulcer, it can be a sign that a resident requires more help than can reasonably be given in your facility. Your staff will be asked to help care for some residents and hopefully heal such ulcers.

What It Is

There are many skin changes that are part of the aging process. Blood flow to the skin decreases with aging, and the skin itself is altered. Lack of mobility, malnutrition, decreased mental alertness, and incontinence of stool or urine increase the chance that a pressure ulcer will develop. All of these factors are more common in the elderly person. Shearing forces result when a resident slides or slips down, with the skin sticking to one surface while the rest of the body moves into another position. Shearing forces block the blood supply to the skin, and contribute to the risk of pressure ulcers.

Pressure ulcers develop because there is pressure over a hard (usually bony) prominence against an external surface. Under normal circumstances, we shift our weight and roll over before the blood supply to our skin and underlying tissues is blocked long enough to cause damage. Any condition that interferes with our normal sensation of discomfort can lead to a pressure ulcer. Residents who are excessively sleepy from sedatives, alcohol, or brain diseases are at increased risk. Skin that is irritated by contact with urine or feces is more likely to develop pressure ulcers. Conditions that interfere with movement, such as Parkinson's disease, multiple sclerosis, and brain or spinal cord injuries also put the resident at risk.

Health Impact

Pressure ulcers can be painful. Infection of the blood from an infected pressure ulcer is fatal in about half of all cases. Drainage from a pressure ulcer contains protein, and large quantities of drainage can contribute to malnutrition. Pressure ulcers heal very slowly and can lead to prolonged periods of illness. This can cause depression and social isolation. Some pressure ulcers develop a foul odor, which contributes to social isolation. Because pressure ulcers often require extensive and expensive nursing care to heal, they can result in the need for hospitalization.

VARIATIONS

Classification and Treatment of Pressure Ulcers

Stage I

Redness over a pressure-bearing area that does not return to normal color within 2 hours after pressure is relieved. This indicates injury to the skin, and may indicate that more damage is present deeper under the skin as well.

Stage I ulcers are often treated with transparent, waterproof films and methods to reduce pressure and prevent further skin damage.

Stage II

Only part of the full thickness of the skin is involved. This often looks like a blister or a very shallow open area of skin. The depth is not much deeper than a sheet of thick paper.

Stage II ulcers are often treated with hydrocolloid dressings, foams, or wet gauze dressings if there are no signs of infection present. If drainage is present, hydrogels or hydrocolloids can be used. Pressure reduction measures are absolutely necessary to allow the ulcer to heal and to prevent others from forming.

Stage III

Full-thickness loss of skin that involves the fatty tissue underneath the skin. The ulcer is a deep crater, with a base that may be red, or have a yellow drainage or even show black, dead tissue.

Stage III ulcers are also treated with foams, hydrocolloid dressings, or wet gauze dressings if there are no signs of infection present. If drainage is present, hydrogels or hydrocolloids can also be used. Often, surgical removal of dead tissue is needed to allow healing. Pressure reduction measures are absolutely necessary to promote healing.

Stage IV

Full-thickness loss of skin that involves the muscles, joints, or bones underneath that area of skin. This is the most serious and difficult-to-heal type of pressure ulcer.

Stage IV ulcers are often treated with surgery to place healthy skin over the damaged area. Hydrogels or alginates can be used to absorb drainage. Stage IV ulcers take prolonged periods of time to heal, and rarely can be managed in a residential care setting without extra help from visiting nurses. Often a resident will need to be transferred to a more intensive level of care.

ALERT

Worsening of confusion, fever, chills, change in alertness, or other major change in condition needs to be reported to the doctor as soon as possible. Remember that infection from pressure sores can spread into the blood and can rapidly become fatal. You must be alert for changes that might signal a new problem.

MEDICATION CHECKLIST

Pressure-Reducing Devices. Thick foam mattresses and special air mattresses, water mattresses, and very specialized electric beds that are inflated with constantly flowing air are useful to reduce pressure and to treat and prevent pressure ulcers. Residential care facilities will rarely care for residents who need anything more elaborate than a thick foam mattress. Much more commonly, soft foam pillows, wheelchair cushions, foam foot protection, and frequent reminders to change position are the type of pressure reduction performed in residential care settings. Do not use doughnut-type devices because they actually increase rather than decrease the risk of pressure ulcers.

Gauze Dressings. These loose mesh cotton gauze dressings are moistened with sterile water or saline (salt water). Do not allow them to fully dry before changing, because that would cause them to adhere to the wound and damage delicate healing tissue.

Films. These clear films mimic the function of intact skin, are waterproof, and can remain in place for 5 to 7 days. They provide no cushioning of the wound. They are generally only used on early or stage I ulcers. Commonly used brands include Opsite and Tegaderm.

Hydrocolloids. These relatively thick dressings stick to the skin by themselves, and interact with fluid in the wound to form a gel that

continued on following page

continued from previous page

protects the wound. They can remain in place for 5 to 7 days. They are used for stage II or III ulcers if no infection is present. Commonly used brands include Duoderm, Tegasorb, and Comfeel.

Foams. These foams are available in spray form, and maintain a moist wound environment to promote healing. They require a cover wrap or dressing to prevent them from falling out of the ulcer. They are used for noninfected stage II or III ulcers. Commonly used brands include Allevyn, LYO foam, and others.

Hydrogels. These gels absorb drainage and require a cover wrap or dressing to prevent them from drying out. They are used for stage II, III, or IV ulcers. Commonly used brands include Vigilon, Carrington gel, and others.

Alginates. These dressings are made from seaweed, absorb drainage very well, and require a cover wrap or dressing to prevent them from drying out. They are used for stage III or IV ulcers. Commonly used brands include Kaltostat, Sorbsan, and others.

YOUR ROLE

Pressure ulcers are not always preventable, but in many cases they could be prevented with frequent turning of a resident, extra nutritional support, and pressure-reducing devices. This level of care may not be easy or even appropriate to provide in the residential care setting. If pressure sores develop in one of your residents, there must be a careful re-evaluation as to whether the resident will need to be transferred to a higher level of care. Many lawsuits are based on residential care facilities and staff attempting to provide more care than they are capable of. Unless you are confident that you can provide the needed care, ask the doctor about proper placement for your resident.

If pressure ulcers are a common occurence in your facility, you need to evaluate the care you are providing to see if it needs improvement. For example, you may be accepting residents who are too sick for you to care for properly, or you may be keeping them too long as they become more frail. Pressure sores require a great deal of staff time, and it may just be impractical to keep residents who need this level of care.

If you do decide that you can care for a resident while trying to help treat a pressure ulcer, then get all the help you need from the doctor and visiting nurses. Frequently have the pressure ulcers checked by a professional to monitor healing, and if the ulcer is not healing as quickly as expected, re-evaluate your ability to provide this type of care.

Make your facility as skin-friendly as possible. Offer skin moisturizer to those with dry skin, and moisture barrier creams to protect the skin of those who are incontinent. Instruct your staff to report any skin problems promptly. Avoid the use of any home remedies to try and heal pressure ulcers.

Medical Treatment

- Surgically cleaning out dead tissue and scars in the ulcer to allow healing to occur
- Surgery to remove or cover over the ulcer
- Prescribing a course of therapy to heal the ulcer, which can include pressure-relieving devices, dressings, antibiotics, and many other treatments
- Treatment to correct problems that contribute to pressure ulcers forming, including poor nutrition, anemia, incontinence, and lack of mobility

Residential Care Actions

- Teach staff to inspect for pressure ulcers when assisting residents with bathing or personal care.
- Report any pressure ulcers promptly to the doctor.
- Report weight loss or any change in level of mobility to the doctor.
- Provide only the skin care prescribed by doctor or nurse for care of the pressure ulcer. Do not use home remedies.
- Report changes in condition of residents that have skin ulcers promptly. They may have infections related to the ulcers.
- Recognize that many residents with skin ulcers will require skilled nursing care to heal the ulcers. You need to position and frequently turn immobile residents. A skin ulcer that is not healing or is getting worse is a sign that you may not be able to safely care for this resident.

 DIET TIPS

- Food should be appetizing and nutritious.
- Offer juice or other beverages between meals.
- Offer dietary supplements or small, frequent meals if appetite is poor.
- Alcohol use should be avoided.

FOR YOUR RECORDS

Health History
- Alcohol use
- Sedative use
- Dementia
- Previous pressure ulcers
- Malnutrition
- Stroke, spinal cord injury, multiple sclerosis, or other neurologic illness

Current Needs
- Weight monitoring
- Monitoring of skin condition, alertness, mobility, urinary or fecal incontinence

COMMON QUESTIONS

How do you change a dressing?
Visiting nurses are often available to inspect healing pressure ulcers and change dressings, but it may be requested that your staff assist in this task. Ask to be instructed as to the proper technique to change the dressing, and ask for written instructions. Wash your hands before and after each dressing change. Disposable gloves or a small plastic sandwich bag can be used to grasp the dressing. The dressing is disposed of in a sealed bag. If you use gloves, throw them away after each dressing change. Do not use the same gloves for more than one resident.

When is a pressure ulcer too severe to be cared for in a residential care facility?
In general, this will depend on your particular facility. Any resident that requires frequent turning is not likely to be able to be safely cared for in a residential care facility. Remember, frequent turning includes the entire night, which is the time that your staff is unlikely to be able to handle this need. In situations where the resident needs complicated care or frequent turning, the resident will need to be transferred to a facility that can handle such residents. If new pressure ulcers are forming under your care, consider them a sign that you cannot handle this particular resident.

Where can I get more information?
The federal government has put together useful information on treating and preventing pressure ulcers. Ask for a copy of *Preventing Pressure Ulcers: Resident Guide*. To order, call toll-free 800-358-9295.

PSYCHIATRIC DISORDERS

Psychiatric disorders affect the brain, which controls thinking ability, mood, appetite, and sleeping. Rather than causing physical changes like cancer or a stroke, psychiatric disorders produce changes in the way a person thinks and/or behaves.

What It Is

Psychiatric disorders are extremely common in residential care residents. In particular, depression becomes more common with aging. People unable to live independently are much more likely to develop depression compared to healthier persons. There are many causes of psychiatric illnesses, and in many cases the cause of the illness is unknown. Heredity plays an important role, and in particular depression and manic-depressive illness tend to run in families. Psychiatric illness can follow an injury to the brain from a disease process such as Parkinson's disease or stroke. The role of life experiences and environment is controversial, but clearly sad events in life can trigger depression. Substance abuse also plays a role, and psychiatric illness itself can contribute to alcohol and drug abuse as a result of self-medication.

Health Impact

Psychiatric disorders can cause many different problems, depending on the particular disease. Some change a person's mood. Depression makes one uncontrollably sad and unable to find pleasure in life. Mania can lead to inappropriately happy and energetic behavior that can be destructive. Anxiety disorders cause feelings of extreme nervousness, and other psychiatric illnesses alter the logical way a person usually thinks. Schizophrenia causes a person to think things are happening that are not. Panic disorders cause sudden waves of nervousness that are uncontrollable without medication.

Any of these disorders can seriously interfere with a person's life. For example, the sadness of depression can lead to suicide attempts. Any psychiatric disorder can interfere with appetite, leading to weight loss and poor nutrition. Sleep also may be disturbed, and relationships with other people can suffer, leading to family discord and severe isolation.

Generally, having a psychiatric illness has a similar meaning to having a lifelong medical illness such as diabetes or arthritis. Psychiatric illnesses usually respond very well to treatment, which might include counseling, drugs, or other forms of therapy. Often, these treatments are needed for many months or even for the rest of the person's life. Just as insulin can control the problems associated with diabetes, medications may be needed to control the problems of depression or schizophrenia. But just as in diabetes, these medications may need to be adjusted periodically. If properly controlled by treatment, the person with a psychiatric disorder can lead a productive and satisfying life.

VARIATIONS

Depression
- Sadness
- Loss of appetite
- Difficulty sleeping or being too sleepy
- Loss of interest in daily events
- Crying
- Loss of pleasure from things that previously were pleasurable
- Loss of desire to live

Psychosis (Schizophrenia)
- Hallucinations (hearing voices or seeing things that are not there)
- Paranoia (inappropriately thinking people are "out to get you")
- Inability to sustain a logical train of thought

Anxiety
- Inappropriate or excessive worry
- Excessive nervousness
- Persistent thoughts that will not go away

ALERT

Anytime a resident relates thoughts of suicide, report it to a doctor immediately. Most suicides are preceded by just this type of warning.

MEDICATION CHECKLIST

Antidepressant Drugs. These drugs can lessen the sadness and loss of interest in life that occur in depression. Common examples include desipramine, nortriptyline (Pamelor), fluoxetine (Prozac), sertraline (Zoloft), and others.

continued on following page

continued from previous page

Antipsychotic Drugs. These drugs are used to treat schizophrenia and cases of depression or dementia in which symptoms of disordered thinking occur. Common examples include haloperidol (Haldol), thioridazine (Mellaril), thiothixine (Navane), and others.

Lithium. This drug can prevent the development of mania (excess energy, inability to sleep, disordered thoughts). Lithium can cause severe side-effects when too much is taken, and frequent blood tests are used to make sure the current dose is correct.

Anti-anxiety Drugs. These drugs calm excess feelings of nervousness. Often, they are also sedating. Common examples are lorazepam (Ativan), diazepam (Valium), oxazepam (Serax), and alprazolam (Xanax). These drugs cause unpleasant withdrawal symptoms when discontinued and should not be stopped abruptly without informing the doctor. Another anti-anxiety drug, buspirone (Buspar), is less sedating and lacks withdrawal effects, but takes several weeks to work.

YOUR ROLE

Many people are not well-informed about psychiatric illness, and terms like "crazy" or "nuts" may be used to describe what is a very real and manageable illness. You need to help the resident with a psychiatric disorder to live with the problem. This will include promoting socialization with other residents, monitoring medications, and observing for side-effects. You are in a position to be the first to notice an important change in behavior or even suicidal thoughts, which need to be communicated as soon as possible to the doctor. The resident should have both a psychiatrist and a primary care doctor. You should discuss with them who should be contacted and what symptoms they want reported.

Medical Treatment
- Counseling and other forms of psychotherapy
- Medications to treat the disorder or help control symptoms
- Psychiatric hospitalization

DIET TIPS

- "Favorite foods" can help cheer up a depressed resident. Family may be able to help you or even prepare some of these dishes.
- Dietary supplements or small, frequent meals can be offered if appetite is poor.
- Certain antidepressant medicines require a special diet. These medications, called *MAO inhibitors,* can cause dangerous symptoms if taken with walnuts, aged cheeses, and certain other foods. If a resident is taking one of these, be certain to obtain very specific information about dietary restrictions.
- Alcohol use should be avoided. Psychiatric medications and alcohol can produce potentially dangerous interactions.

FOR YOUR RECORDS

Health History
- Previous psychiatric illness, hospitalization, and/or suicide attempts
- Medication use
- Alcohol use

Current Needs
- Weight monitoring
- Sensitivity to usual mood
- Observation for changes in normal sleep pattern
- Recognition of and treatment for disordered thoughts

COMMON QUESTIONS

A resident thinks someone is poisoning him, and refuses to eat or take his medication. What should I do?
Fear that someone intends to harm you can be a symptom of a psychiatric disorder. This situation should be referred to the resident's doctor immediately.

The resident is old and very sick. Isn't it normal for him or her to be depressed?
Depression is never normal. Even after losing a spouse or after a major illness, it is normal to bounce back. We know that depres-

sion responds very well to treatment. Since we can make even very frail or sick people feel better by treating depression, it is important to notify the doctor when you suspect depression so treatment can be started.

Can a person who has been treated for a psychiatric disorder ever stop taking medication safely?

In many cases it is possible to stop medication without the problem returning. However, this should never be done without discussion with the doctor first. Some people have failed many efforts at stopping the medication in the past, and will predictably get very sick if medication is stopped without medical supervision.

RASH

A rash is a visible change in the appearance of the skin and may include redness, either throughout the skin or in dots or patches.

With age the skin becomes thinner, dryer, and more prone to injury.

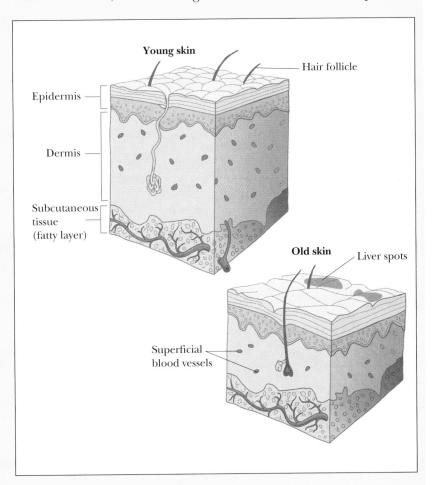

What It Is   The skin is the largest organ of the body and is served by numerous tiny blood vessels. When an infection or inflammation is present in the skin, more blood flows into these vessels, and we see a reddish color to the skin. Sometimes the body fights a disease by forming pus—a collection of dead white blood cells. This pus can be visible in the skin as white raised bumps. A rash is a signal that may warn of an allergy, infection, internal cancer, or contact with an irritating substance such as urine. Generally, a new rash requires medical attention.

One of the most common causes of rash in older persons is simple dry skin: the dry skin is itchy, the resident scratches, and a rash develops!

Another common cause is skin infection, which may be caused by bacteria, viruses, or funguses. Each produces a particular pattern of rash.

Sunburn also produces a rash. Soaking in urine can cause a rash. Areas of the body where sweat collects, such as under the breasts or in the groin, can become infected with a fungus. Some internal cancers produce a rash, and a rash is a common symptom of allergy to a drug, as discussed in Section IV.

Health Impact

Rashes can be very uncomfortable, painful, and itchy. They can be associated with a fever or general bad feeling. Other rashes can be completely pain free and, in fact, the resident is unaware of the rash. If a rash causes pain or itching, the resident may not be able to sleep well. The rash may be so uncomfortable that the resident's appetite is affected. In severe cases, a resident can become mentally confused because of severe itchiness and discomfort.

VARIATIONS

Minor or Mild Rashes

Some rashes will not bother the resident or may cause only minor annoyance. The following can be present:

- Itching
- Tingling
- Redness
- "Dots"
- Swollen bumps
- Raised blisters

Severe Rashes

- A rash that spreads over the entire body causing fever, severe itching, or pain
- Blisters that are localized to one part of the body and cause severe pain, tingling, or fever
- A rash that starts as or develops into a raised, red, tender area that spreads over hours or days
- A rash with large blisters that break and cause weeping or oozing of fluid

Potential Problems or Complications

- Infection that spreads to the bloodstream—called *sepsis* or *blood poisoning*
- Scarring
- Persistent pain (can occur after the rash of shingles)

ALERT

Contact the appropriate doctors if a rash seems to be spreading among your residents. You may have an infectious rash spreading through your facility. Also be sensitive to the possibility of a rash developing as a reaction to an over-the-counter medication being used to treat a rash, and consult the doctor with any questions.

MEDICATION CHECKLIST

Skin Moisturizers. Lotions and creams help trap moisture in the skin and help treat the dry skin that is a common cause of rash. They are best used immediately after bathing.

Steroids. Steriods are strong anti-inflammatory drugs that reduce the inflammation that causes rashes. They are usually applied as creams, lotions, or ointments, but can be given as pills, shots, or injected directly into the rash by the doctor. Common examples are triamcinolone (TAC) and hydrocortisone (HC).

Antibiotics. Antibiotics are used to treat bacterial infections that cause a rash to appear. They can be given orally or applied as a cream or ointment. Common examples include cephalexin (Keflex), which can be taken by mouth, and triple antibiotic cream (Neosporin), which is applied directly to the rash.

Antifungal Drugs. Antifungal drugs treat rashes caused by fungal infections. They can be taken orally or applied as a cream or ointment. Common examples include griseofulvin, taken by mouth, and nystatin powder (Mycostatin), applied directly to the rash.

Antiviral Drugs. Antiviral drugs treat rashes caused by viral infections. They can be taken orally or applied as a cream or ointment. Common examples include acyclovir (Zovirax), which can be taken by mouth or applied as an ointment.

YOUR ROLE

You can provide an environment that will help minimize rashes by encouraging frequent toileting for residents who might otherwise be incontinent during the day. Your staff might need to change these residents' clothes and diapers more frequently. Avoid excessively hot water for bathing, and provide skin moisturizers. If a rash develops, promptly obtain medical attention for the affected resident(s). If scabies or other insect problems develop in your facility, make sure they are thoroughly eliminated.

Medical Treatment
- Skin moisturizers
- Medication to help reduce itching or treat underlying illness, such as infection
- Creams or ointments to soothe the rash or treat infection

 DIET TIPS

- Note any food allergies.
- Severe rashes can cause loss of body fluid from weeping blisters and extra sweating. Make sure a resident with a rash drinks plenty of fluids.

FOR YOUR RECORDS

Health History
- Previous rashes
- Medication use
- Previous allergies to medications, detergents, foods, etc.
- Previous shingles

Current Needs
- Relief of dry skin, itchiness, or moisture under breasts or in groin
- Preventive or care measures for urinary incontinence

COMMON QUESTIONS

Are shingles contagious?
Shingles is a rash caused by the same virus that causes chicken pox. Years and even decades after having chicken pox, the virus

can become active again and the rash of shingles can develop. You cannot catch shingles from contact with this rash, but persons who have not had chicken pox can catch it from someone with shingles. This can be a problem for your staff as well as for other residents.

What is scabies?
Scabies is an infection caused by a tiny spider-like insect called a mite. The infection is easily spread by contact with the rash or with bedding or clothing of the affected resident. Staff members and other residents can develop scabies at the same time. Scabies should be treated with medication as soon as it is reported to the resident's doctor. Other treatment measures include laundering all the clothing and bedding of affected residents in very hot water at the same time.

How can you prevent dry skin from becoming a rash?
Hot water dries skin more than cooler water does. Encourage residents with dry skin to avoid steaming hot showers or baths. Use moisturizing lotions after bathing. Many soaps are very drying. Ask the doctor which soap to use for a resident with dry skin problems.

How can you prevent rashes when the resident is incontinent?
Changing a resident's garments as frequently as possible will help avoid unnecessary contact of urine with the skin. Special creams, called moisture barrier creams, can also help protect skin.

SENSORY IMPAIRMENTS

Sensory impairments include a reduction or loss of vision, hearing, smell, taste, balance, or touch.

What It Is

Some changes in the eyes, ears, and other sensory organs occur as a normal part of aging. Other changes may occur because of a disease process.

- Blindness or severe visual impairment can be caused by diabetes, glaucoma, blood clots in the eyes, or degeneration of the nerves of the eye.
- Hearing impairment is more often due to age changes, but factors like the buildup of ear wax play a role.
- The senses of smell, taste, and balance all decrease with age, but injury, stroke, or medication side-effects can also cause problems.

Health Impact

Poor vision and hearing can lead to social isolation and withdrawal from usual daily activities, which can lead to depression. An inability to participate in conversations, to read a newspaper, or watch television can cause a resident to feel out of touch and can actually produce what may appear to be signs of dementia. Impairment of the senses of smell and taste can cause a resident to be unable to detect smoke from a fire or the smell of spoiled food. The appetite can be poor because food does not taste good. Poor balance can contribute to falls, and in particular makes it hard for a resident to catch himself or herself after a stumble.

Many of your residents will have poor function of one or more senses, and you can help by adapting your facility for specific problems. Many organizations in your community should be able to help. For example, the telephone company may offer free or low-cost special equipment to improve communication abilities. The library can help you get books on tape and large print books for residents with poor vision. Ask the resident's doctor if anything can be done to help the resident. This might be a medical treatment or an assistive device to help the resident live more safely and comfortably with the limitation.

VARIATIONS

Early Symptoms

- Difficulty with night vision
- Occasionally missing a word in conversation

Advanced Symptoms
- Inability to drive due to poor vision
- Inability to read normal size print
- Complaints from other residents about television or radio being too loud

Potential Problems and Complications
- Withdrawal
- Depression
- Frequent falls

ALERT

Any sudden loss of sensory function should be treated as an emergency—contact the doctor immediately.

MEDICATION CHECKLIST

Eye Drops. These can be used to treat glaucoma and other eye disorders. Common examples are pilocarpine, timolol (Timoptic), and others.

Ear Drops. These can soften ear wax and help the doctor remove wax that interferes with hearing. An example is carbanide peroxide (Debrox).

YOUR ROLE

Make the facility as brightly lit as possible. Get any assistive devices like magnifiers, telephone amplifiers. Use carpeting and wall hangings to help absorb echoes. Make sure residents use hearing aids when they have them, and teach your staff how to change the batteries and manage the hearing aid for residents who need assitance. Use spices and flavorful foods to help compensate for losses in taste and smell. Additional measures include a quiet and non-distracting environment, large print books and newspapers, and earphones for television and radio use.

Medical Treatment
- Glasses
- Hearing aids
- Cleaning out ear wax

- Cataract and other eye surgeries
- Eye drops

 DIET TIPS

- Use special diets like low sodium (salt) only if prescribed by doctor.
- Fresh fruits and vegetables usually have much more flavor and smell compared to processed foods.
- To help keep diet as flavorful as possible, use spices and herbs.
- Offer dietary supplements or small, frequent meals if appetite is poor.
- Alcohol use should be avoided in residents with poor balance or vision.

FOR YOUR RECORDS

Health History
- Previous vision or hearing problems
- Previous falls
- Medication use

Current Needs
- Weight and appetite monitoring
- Use of assistive/corrective devices
- Recognition of depression

COMMON QUESTIONS

Can cataracts be treated with a laser?
No. Laser technology can be used, however, for certain problems that develop a few months after cataract surgery in some residents. The only way to remove cataracts now is surgery.

Why does the resident not wear his or her hearing aid?
Hearing aids do not make hearing normal in the way that glasses sometimes improve eyesight. Hearing aids make all noises louder, and may prove disturbing in noisy rooms. Hearing aids also require maintenance and proper care; the batteries need to be changed frequently, the hearing aid needs to be correctly insert-

ed, and the tubing needs to be free of wax. If a resident is not using a hearing aid, contact the audiologist who dispensed the hearing aid or the doctor, and find out what can be done.

The resident's balance seems to be getting worse. What can be done?
A change in balance can be a drug side-effect or a sign that a stroke has occurred. If you notice a change in the resident's balance, contact the doctor.

SHORTNESS OF BREATH

Shortness of breath is a feeling of not being able to get enough air while breathing.

What It Is

The heart and lungs work together to maintain an adequate supply of oxygen circulating to all body cells. The lungs pass oxygen from the air into the blood and remove excess carbon dioxide with each exhale. The heart then pumps the oxygen-carrying blood to all the vital areas of the body. Any impairment of either the lungs or the heart can produce the feeling of shortness of breath.

Shortness of breath can be caused by a variety of circumstances, including being out of shape, pneumonia, asthma, blood clots in the lungs, lung cancer, or a food that is accidentally inhaled into the lungs. Perhaps the most common cause of chronic shortness of breath is damage from smoking. Two common diseases, emphysema and chronic bronchitis, are both related to smoking.

Congestive heart failure causes salty fluid to build up in the lungs, which can cause mild or even severe shortness of breath, or difficulty breathing that develops suddenly at night, causing the resident to wake up, desperately short of breath.

Health Impact

The feeling of being winded or out of breath is usually worse when doing something physical, such as walking, carrying things, and talking. Shortness of breath may cause a resident to stop doing things for himself or herself, stop activities like walking or bathing, and stop carrying on conversations with staff and other residents. Confusion and sleepiness also may be associated with shortness of breath, and if breathing difficulties are long-lasting, a resident may become withdrawn and depressed.

Shortness of breath can be a sign of a new illness, like pneumonia or congestive heart failure. If a resident who is not usually short of breath becomes short of breath, contact a doctor immediately.

A resident may need to use oxygen to relieve shortness of breath that does not fully respond to medical treatment. These residents are extremely vulnerable to heart and lung problems. If shortness of breath becomes more severe than usual, contact the resident's doctor.

VARIATIONS

Early Symptoms
- Shortness of breath with exercise
- Nervousness
- Fatigue
- Increased heart rates with exercise

Advanced Symptoms
- Shortness of breath at rest
- Feeling of suffocation during sleep
- Swelling of the lower legs and feet
- Wheezing
- Cough
- Blue tint to skin

Potential Problems and Complications
- Shortness of breath even with supplemental oxygen
- Sudden death

ALERT

Sudden shortness of breath, especially shortness of breath at rest, is a medical emergency. Contact the doctor immediately.

MEDICATION CHECKLIST

Bronchodilators. These drugs open up the breathing tubes in the lungs. Some can have the side-effect of making the heart beat too fast, especially if the medication is used in excess. Bronchodilators can be given in pill form, but most often they are used in inhalers (commonly called puffers). Examples include albuterol (Ventolin, Proventil) and ipratropium (Atrovent).

Steroids. These drugs reduce inflammation in the breathing tubes of the lungs. Although they can be given in pill form (most often as prednisone), more often they are used in inhalers or puffers. Examples include Azmacort and Vanceril.

Diuretics. Commonly called water pills, diuretics actually help eliminate excess salt *and* water. They can limit the swelling of the legs and the collection of salty water in the lungs. Common examples include furosemide (Lasix), hydrochlorothiazide, and triamterene/hydrochlorothiazide (Dyazide).

YOUR ROLE

Residents who develop shortness of breath may have pneumonia or another serious medical illness. You must help them get medical attention as soon as possible. Residents with conditions that leave them permanently short of breath will need your help supervising medications. They will be very sensitive to colds, flu, and other lung infections, and you will need to contact the doctor if they seem more short of breath than usual. Residents who need oxygen all the time may feel isolated. You will need to help them socialize, and you may need to ask the doctor about portable oxygen to help them leave the facility for social visits and doctor's appointments.

Medical Treatment
- X-ray tests and other diagnostic procedures to determine the cause
- Diuretics (water pills) to remove excess fluid from the lungs
- Medication to help breathing
- Antibiotics to treat infections
- Inhalers—small canisters of medicine used to puff doses of medicine into the lungs
- Oxygen
- Hospitalization

 DIET TIPS

- Low-sodium (salt) diet is often prescribed by doctor if congestive heart failure is present.
- Dietary supplements or small, frequent meals should be offered if appetite is poor.
- Special diets are sometimes prescribed in cases of severe lung disease.
- Alcohol use should be avoided.

FOR YOUR RECORDS

Health History
- Previous heart attack
- High blood pressure
- Previous or current tobacco use
- Asthma
- Medication use
- Alcohol use

Current Needs
- Weight monitoring
- Extra pillows to aid breathing during sleep
- Preventive or care measures for urinary incontinence
- Sodium (salt) restricted diet if prescribed
- Elastic stockings to improve circulation in the legs
- Elevating the legs to reduce swelling
- Supervision of medication and oxygen use
- Discouraging cigarette smoking

COMMON QUESTIONS

How serious is shortness of breath that happens only during exercise?
It can be very serious, as it may represent the first sign of a lung or heart disease. This is the best time to treat most diseases, so it is very important to bring this problem to the attention of a doctor.

The resident already is very short of breath from emphysema. Is there any benefit from stopping smoking at this point?
Absolutely. Although the problems with breathing may not completely go away, breathing should improve if smoking is stopped.

What level of activity is appropriate for the resident who has shortness of breath?
Some residents get short of breath from walking or other mild exercise because they are out of shape and would benefit from regular exercise. Other residents may be short of breath because of lung or heart disease and may get worse or even faint if forced to exercise. Because each resident is different, you will need to discuss any questions or problems with the doctor.

STROKE

Stroke is the term used to describe a variety of conditions that cause a disruption in normal blood flow to the brain.

What It Is

Each area of the brain has a specific function. For example, one area instructs the muscles to move in the right arm, and other areas are responsible for speech, balance, vision, and the sense of touch.

Blood flow to the brain can be interrupted by a blood clot in the blood vessels leading to the brain, by a blood clot traveling from the heart and lodging in the brain, or when a blood vessel in the brain bursts, spilling blood directly into the brain. Factors that increase the risk of stroke include high blood pressure, diabetes, or a type of irregular heart beat called *atrial fibrillation.*

When blood flow to an area of the brain is interrupted, functions controlled by that region are lost. Symptoms may include:

Functions affected by stroke correspond to area of brain deprived of oxygen.

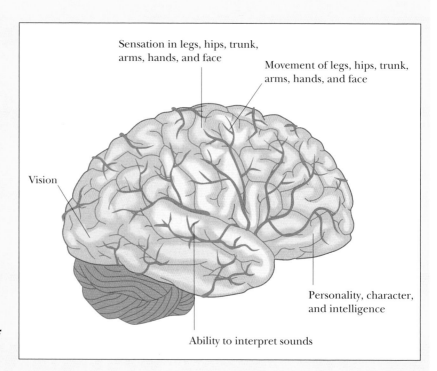

Sensation in legs, hips, trunk, arms, hands, and face

Movement of legs, hips, trunk, arms, hands, and face

Vision

Personality, character, and intelligence

Ability to interpret sounds

- Weakness or paralysis of the face, arm, and/or leg on one side of the body
- Slurred speech or inability to find the right words
- Coughing when attempting to swallow
- Unconsciousness immediately after a stroke

Unfortunately, brain tissue does not heal in the same way that skin heals after an injury, and after a stroke there is permanent loss of brain tissue. Sometimes the remaining healthy brain tissue can take over new jobs and the individual recovers lost function, but often the loss of function is permanent. Rehabilitation emphasizes achieving the highest possible level of recovery and adjustment to, or methods to compensate for, permanently lost functions.

Health Impact

Stroke is a medical emergency that requires hospitalization to control brain swelling and to permit continuous observation. Often, the seriousness of a stroke and its long-term outcome cannot be determined for several days while the individual's condition stabilizes. During this period certain additional problems like urinary incontinence, difficulty swallowing, constipation, depression, and painful shoulders or hands may become evident and require additional treatment.

VARIATIONS

Symptoms

- Sudden weakness of one side of the body or loss of speech or vision
- Sudden loss of consciousness or uncontrollable sleepiness
- Sudden and severe headache

Long-Term Problems and Complications

- Persistent problems with speech, sight, or muscle strength on the affected side
- Difficulty swallowing
- Tightness of the muscles on paralyzed side
- Urinary incontinence
- Severe tightness of joints on paralyzed side, called *contractures*
- Changes in behavior, with periods of depression or impairment in judgment or memory
- Frequent bladder infections
- Constipation

ALERT

The new onset of weakness of one part of the body, loss of speech, or severe sleepiness of a resident needs to be reported to the doctor immediately.

MEDICATION CHECKLIST

There are no drugs currently available to *reverse* the damage done by strokes or to limit the damage of a stroke as it happens; however, certain types of medications may be part of a resident's long-term care.

Aspirin. In low, daily doses, aspirin can make the blood less "sticky" and therefore less likely to form clots. Many doctors prescribe a low dose of aspirin daily to prevent strokes.

Seizure Medications. After a stroke, many residents develop epilepsy (seizures) and medications are prescribed to reduce the frequency and severity of seizures. Specific types are discussed in the section on seizures.

YOUR ROLE

A new stroke is an emergency and needs to be reported to the doctor immediately. After a stroke, the resident may need extra help with many daily activities. For example, the resident may need help cutting foods into small pieces, as well as help with dressing, bathing, and toilet transfers. Safety can be helped by eliminating exposed carpet edges and electrical cords to prevent tripping, and by installing handrails and elevated toilet seats in the bathroom. Communication may be impaired by slurred speech or loss of ability to produce speech. If you think the problems of a particular resident make it difficult or unsafe to meet specific needs in your facility, alternative care or living arrangements should be arranged.

Rehabilitation from a stroke may be continued while a person is living in your facility. Physical therapists help strengthen muscles and improve balance. They teach the resident to use mechanical aids such as walkers and canes. Speech and language therapists help improve the damaged speech. Occupational therapists help improve skills such as washing and dressing, and may help with swallowing problems.

If a resident is able to return to your facility, you will be involved in coordinating care by professionals involved in rehabilitation and can play a vital role in helping the resident learn to live with any residual problems left from the stroke, such as learning to live with a paralyzed side. In addition, measures to prevent future strokes will be needed, such as the use of blood thinners or closer monitoring of efforts to control high blood pressure.

Medical Treatment

- Blood thinners to prevent future strokes
- Rehabilitation to help recover lost function
- Assistive devices such as canes, wheelchairs, special beds, grasping devices, etc.
- Sodium (salt) restricted diet if hypertension is present
- Special consistency diets (e.g., thickened liquids) if swallowing impairment is present
- Skin care and massage for paralyzed limbs
- Moving weak or paralyzed joints through their range of motion
- Measures to prevent constipation

DIET TIPS

- Low-sodium (salt) diet may be prescribed by doctor.
- Special consistency foods (soft, no thin liquids, etc.) may be prescribed by doctor.
- Extra fiber can be given if constipation present.
- Dietary supplements or small, frequent meals can be offered if appetite is poor.
- If part of meal is ignored, food may need to be rearranged during meal so resident notices it.
- Alcohol use should be avoided.

FOR YOUR RECORDS

Health History

- Previous strokes, high blood pressure, or constipation
- Difficulties swallowing
- Medication use

- Alcohol use
- Nutritional problems

Current Needs
- Weight monitoring
- Skin care
- Special diet
- Activity restrictions
- Use of assistive devices (canes, walker, etc.)
- Assistance in managing urinary and/or fecal incontinence

COMMON QUESTIONS

How long does it take to recover from a stroke?
Some people are lucky enough to have full recovery of function after a stroke, but most are left with some permanent impairment. Fortunately, there is often improvement in function in the first few days after the stroke, as brain tissue swelling subsides and healing of damaged but not destroyed brain tissue begins. This improvement can continue for as long as six months or even a year after the stroke.

Why do some residents ignore part of their food or not wash part of their body?
One possible loss that occurs when brain tissue is destroyed is the awareness of part of the body (often the whole left or right side). A resident with such a problem will not recognize food on one half of the plate. If the plate is rotated so that the food is on the opposite side of the plate, they will then finish it. Or a person may not realize that one arm belongs to his or her body and may not shave or wash half the face. Such residents require extra supervision with meals and personal care.

How much activity is appropriate for the resident?
Given the many different possibilities for problems related to a stroke, the best level of activity for each person should be discussed with the doctor. In general, it is good to encourage exercise and independence for persons recovering from a stroke. In some cases, however, the resident's judgment is poor, and he or she may attempt inappropriate or dangerous activities. When doubt about safety exists, always ask for medical guidance.

WEAKNESS OR NUMBNESS

The sudden development of weakness or numbness of one side of the body can be a sign of a stroke, a severely pinched nerve, or other serious medical problems. After the immediate problem is treated, permanent weakness or numbness may persist. Such people may have special needs in residential care.

What It Is

The brain controls muscle function and the sense of touch throughout the body. The signals connecting the brain to the rest of the body are carried by nerves. You can think of nerves as the electrical wiring of the body. Just as a television will stop working if you pull the plug, the muscle strength and sense of touch in part of the body will shut off if the part of the brain or the nerve that supplies it is damaged. Sometimes the muscle itself is affected by a disease, and then weakness occurs without any numbness. Symptoms may include:

* Weakness, numbness, or paralysis of the face, arm, and/or leg on *one* side of the body
* Numbness of *both* hands and *both* feet, with normal sensation in the center of the body

Weakness of the whole body, without one part of the body being affected more than any other, can be caused by many different medical conditions, as well as from drugs and psychological problems such as depression.

A resident with weakness may not complain about it but you may notice that the resident drops objects, stumbles, falls, uses the hands to push off the arms of a chair to get up, or grasps your arm for help to transfer out of bed or a chair. A resident may stop activities he or she was formerly able to do unassisted, such as shave, comb his or her hair, or brush the teeth. If the weakness affects face muscles, facial expressions may be distorted.

The new onset of numbness or weakness may be due to a stroke or blood clot pressing on the brain. This will require immediate notification of the doctor and in most cases transfer to an emergency room. Slow development of weakness or numbness over months or years can be the result of diabetes, thyroid disease, and other medical conditions.

Health Impact   Unless weakness or numbness can be reversed with medical treatment, the resident will have to live with this problem indefinitely. Weakness of an arm or leg can make such common activities as walking, dressing, and feeding oneself difficult or impossible without help. Numbness can prevent a resident from noticing minor cuts and other injuries, so that infection or large skin ulcers can form, putting the resident at risk for limb amputation.

VARIATIONS

Early Symptoms
- Sudden weakness or numbness of one side
- Slow development of weakness of one or more parts of the body
- Slow development of numbness or tingling in the hands and feet
- Persistent problems with speech, sight, or muscle strength on the affected side
- Tightness of the muscles on the paralyzed side
- Frequent small cuts and injuries to the hands and feet due to clumsiness
- Frequent falls

Potential Problems and Complications
- Severe tightness of joints on paralyzed side, called *contractures*
- Frequent skin infections or skin ulcers in numb areas
- Loss of ability to walk

ALERT

Any new onset of weakness or numbness of one part of the body needs to be reported to the doctor immediately.

MEDICATION CHECKLIST

If medical problems such as high blood pressure or diabetes contribute to the weakness or numbness, then medication can be used to help treat these conditions. However, there are no medications that are commonly given to treat the weakness or numbness alone.

YOUR ROLE

A new stroke is an emergency and needs to be reported to the doctor immediately. After a stroke, permanent weakness may make the resident need extra help with many activities of daily living. If you think the problems of a particular resident make caring for him or her impossible or unsafe in your facility, alternative care or living arrangements may have to be arranged.

When numbness is present the resident will need to examine his or her feet and other numb areas to watch for cuts or other injuries. If the resident has poor vision or confusion, you or your staff will need to help with this inspection.

Medical Treatment

- Hospitalization or special tests to identify the cause of the problem
- Blood thinners to prevent stroke
- Rehabilitation to help recover lost function
- Assistive devices such as canes, wheelchairs, special beds, grasping devices

Residential Care Actions

- Safety devices (handrails, firm chairs with arms, railings in the bathrooms, and elevated toilet seats)
- Skin care and massage for paralyzed limbs
- Moving weak or paralyzed joints through their full range of motion
- Elimination of exposed carpet edges and electrical cords to prevent tripping
- Reporting any changes in the resident's condition, such as new weakness, falling, or decreased alertness

DIET TIPS

- A special-consistency diet is often prescribed by the doctor if swallowing is impaired.
- A dietitian may need to teach your staff the correct food for residents with swallowing difficulty.
- Dietary supplements or small, frequent meals may be offered if appetite is poor.
- Special easy-to-handle utensils can help residents with weakness cut their food and feed themselves.
- Some residents with weakness on one side of the body will ignore that side of the plate and food will be left even if the resident is still hungry. Turning the plate around so that the food is on the other side can be helpful.

FOR YOUR RECORDS

Health History
- Previous stroke
- High blood pressure or diabetes
- Difficulty swallowing
- Medication use
- Alcohol use
- Nutritional problems

Current Needs
- Weight and skin condition monitoring
- Special diet
- Assistance with activities of daily living and use of assistive devices (canes, walker, etc.)

COMMON QUESTIONS

Does the weakness or numbness from a stroke get better?
Most of the recovery after a stroke occurs in the days and first few weeks after the stroke. After six months, very little additional recovery of strength is possible. Improvement after that time is from learning to use the unaffected muscles better rather than from increased strength.

What is a pinched nerve?

Nerves travel through the bones of the spine into the body, arms, and legs. Pressure on the nerve at any point can cause weakness or numbness in the part of the body supplied by that nerve. This pinching can be from a *slipped disk*—a jelly-like cushion between spinal bones that can sometimes be damaged and press on nerves. The nerve can be pinched in the wrist, called *carpal tunnel syndrome.* Severe arthritis in the spine can also pinch nerves.

What are specific precautions needed for someone with weakness of one side of the body?

Walking is often difficult if a stroke has caused weakness or paralysis on one side of the body. Residents may require assistance getting into and out of chairs, and with climbing stairs. Handrails in corridors and bathrooms and having sturdy chairs with arms can reduce the risk of falls. Swallowing can be difficult after a stroke if one side of the face is weak, and a special diet may be prescribed that is easier for the resident to swallow. You should always contact the doctor if there is choking or coughing during meals, or if falls are occurring.

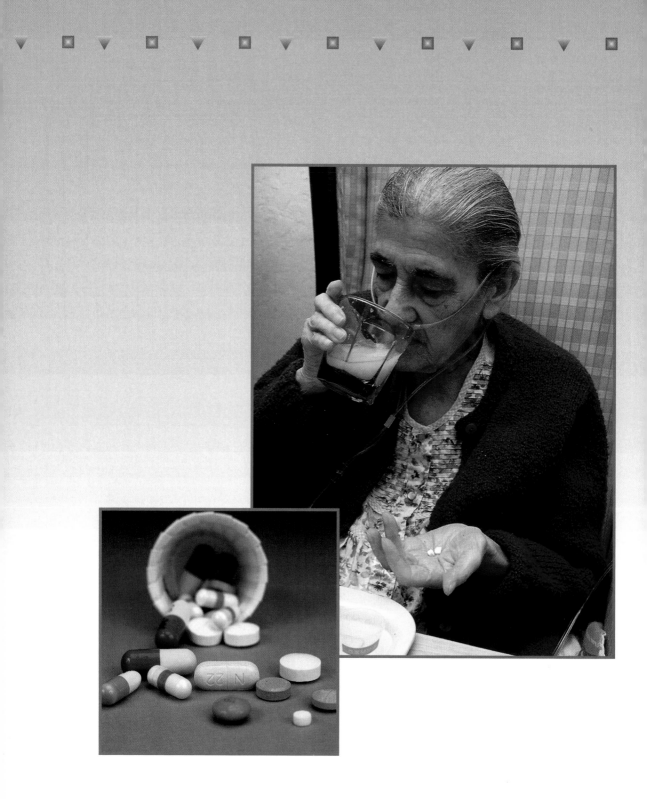

Understanding Medications

YOUR ROLE

Resident needs vary considerably in terms of the level of assistance that managers and caregivers need to provide. Anyone who assists others in taking medications is responsible for their own actions. You should follow the five "rights" of drug administration to prevent any unnecessary mistakes.

- Right drug – Read the label to be sure you have the right drug for the right resident.

- Right dose – Carefully read the instructions on the package label to be sure you give the right amount of a drug.

- Right resident – Be sure you know your residents so you give the right resident the right drug.

- Right route – Check the doctor's orders and the package label.

- Right time – Check the doctor's orders to be sure that you give the drug at the right time.

You should have some understanding of what the drug is being given for and what side-effects or reactions to look for. Remember all residents have the right to refuse medications unless judged to be incompetent by a court of law.

How you prepare yourself to provide for these needs will play a key role in determining how effective you are in administering medications to your residents. The process of ensuring effective drug therapy includes:

- Assurance that residents "rights" are followed

- Follow-up reporting to the prescribing doctor as needed

A detailed description of what needs to be considered in safely helping your residents with medications is provided later in this section. Your responsibilities can be very minimal or can be nearly as involved as nursing facility responsibilities, depending on the needs of residents, staff capabilities, and your own goals. Licensed nurses on staff can administer medications identical to those in nursing facilities if state law permits. The range of services you might offer is listed below:

1. Ordering prescription refills, over the counter medications, and medical supplies from the pharmacy of the resident's choice.

2. Helping resident obtain medications, reminding residents when it is time to take their medications, and ensuring that their medication supplies are reordered as needed and stored properly.

3. Storing resident's medications in a central area, assuming responsibility for obtaining all medications for residents, verifying current directions for use with doctors, providing the right drug and dose at the right time, preparing the dose for the resident's use in a cup or other container, and providing physical assistance as needed (for example, helping a person with shaky hands to hold an eye dropper or a medicine cup).

Some states have laws that make it difficult to provide direct assistance except by a licensed nurse or other licensed health care provider. Be sure to check your state's laws before offering extensive assistance to any resident.

Regardless of the level of service provided, caregivers should be alert for possible drug reactions and for opportunities to help residents with their medications. Sometimes this will require contacting the resident's doctor or pharmacist, but it can be as simple as suggesting that the resident do the same.

HOW MEDICATIONS WORK

Medications are prescribed for a variety of reasons; however, specific benefits can be put into three categories:

Guidelines for Helping with Medications

1. Learn the metric and Apothecary systems of measurement as well as standard abbreviations to help you understand drug strengths and doses (see Appendix 2, Measurement Equivalents, and Appendix 3, Common Abbreviations and Their Meanings).

2. Establish a way to keep track of how doctors want residents to take their medications. Pharmacy labels do not always include the most current directions for use given to a resident when visiting or speaking with their doctor.

3. Establish a good working relationship with at least one pharmacy and one or more pharmacists.

4. Identify how much assistance each resident needs with medications and what assistance is required. This information should be documented (see Figure 4-1, Sample Medication Schedule).

5. Be sure that residents who store their own drugs in their rooms have a safe place that is away from heat, light, and moisture. Bathroom medicine cabinets are not good storage locations for medications that are only taken occasionally. Medications can lose their potency or be altered by changes in temperature and humidity.

6. Establish a simple scheduling method (Figure 4-1) for direct assistance or reminders for medication assistance. This will help when a doctor changes a medication schedule while the resident is still using a medication labeled with previous directions. You may choose to keep a record just for scheduling, as long as local laws do not require the recording of each dose.

7. Use a system to ensure that prescription drugs are reordered in plenty of time, and be sure that the system is efficient. Remember: the easier it is for pharmacies, the more services they will be able to provide for you. A different approach will be needed for medications residents store themselves.

8. Ask your pharmacist to visit occasionally to review your procedures and to meet with residents who may have questions about their medications. It may not be possible to obtain these services without payment in some areas, but it may be well worth the investment.

9. Take the time to write detailed procedures on medication ordering, storage, and administration, including self-administration and administation with assistance.

10. If you have a fairly large facility, and you directly assist a number of residents with their medications, you may be able to have the pharmacy dispense drugs in punch cards. These cards are easy to use and provide you or the resident with a way of telling very quickly if the proper number of doses has been taken and how many remain.

Continued on the following page

Continued from the previous page

11. Medication costs should always be a concern. A pharmacist can quickly provide documentation of drug therapy, especially when residents go to more than one doctor. Most pharmacies maintain "patient profiles" on a computer. These profiles allow the pharmacist to screen for potential interactions, allergies, and other information that is important to your resident.

12. Use a fax machine. Nearly all pharmacies and doctors' offices use fax machines because they offer a fast, effective method of communication. If you obtain instructions from a doctor about a resident's medication that you cannot read (not an uncommon problem), you may be able to fax it to the pharmacy for clarification.

1. To achieve a cure by eliminating all problems associated with a disease

2. To arrest or manage a disease process while not actually curing the problem

3. To treat symptoms

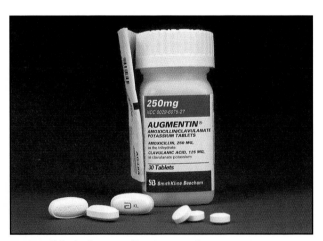

An antibiotic is a medication used to "cure" an infection.

Cures and Replacement Therapy

Very few drugs actually cure a disease. Antibiotics eliminate the cause of an infection. Other drugs replace something the body lacks. In some cases this replacement therapy continues only until the body adjusts to the need. For example thyroid replacement hormone is given because there is a lack of adequate amounts of thyroid produced by the body. Similar examples include treatment of anemia with folic acid, vitamin B_{12}, or iron, each of which is either lacking in the diet or cannot be adequately absorbed by the body. Replacement therapy is either short term or lifelong.

Arresting a Disease Process

Most drug therapy falls into the second category—medications that control the effects of a disease and often slow the process of a disease. Although the results may be favorable (for example, well-controlled high blood pressure), any medication is capable of producing side-effects. Except when there is a change in the body or some other non-drug treatment (such as surgery), this type of therapy is long-term.

Symptomatic Relief

The third category of drug therapy includes drugs such as cough syrups and medications to relieve pain. These drugs are usually used for a relatively short period of time to relieve symptoms but may also be used on a long-term basis to provide comfort.

"As Needed" (PRN)

In the first and second categories it is very important that therapy continue exactly as ordered by the doctor. Even when symptoms disappear, the disease may progress because the underlying problem or cause of the disease continues. Variations in dosing time, if significant, can interfere with the effectiveness of many of these drugs. Many studies have shown that elderly persons are more likely than younger persons to take medications improperly. All too often they end up in hospitals because they failed to take a medication or took it too often. For this reason, assistance with medications is one of the most valuable services your residential care facility can provide.

For drugs that are given short-term to treat symptoms, medications may be scheduled on an "as needed" (PRN) basis. Exact dosing schedules are not as important, because the primary purpose of the therapy is to relieve symptoms and make the person feel better. However, many PRN medications are powerful drugs, and doses should be given exactly as the doctor has ordered. (Always be sure the doctor specifies how frequently a prescription PRN drug may be given, in what dose, and for what reason or symptom.) If a non-prescription (also called "over-the-counter" or OTC) drug is involved, fol-

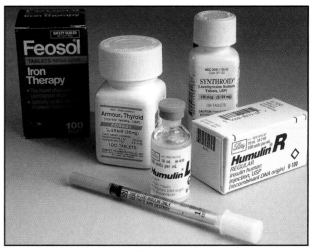

Iron, insulin, and thyroid hormone are examples of drugs used for replacement therapy.

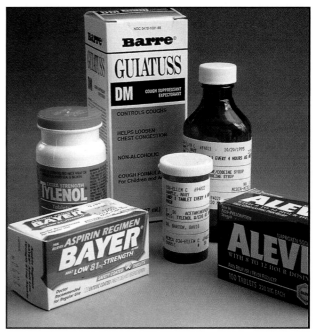

A variety of medications is available over the counter and by prescription for the temporary relief of symptoms.

FIGURE 4-1 SAMPLE MEDICATION SCHEDULE

Sunnyside Medication Schedule

Resident: Jean Allen   **Rm:** 121   **Dr.** Stephens   **Date:** 9/1/96

Level of Assistance, Special Instructions: All but artificial tears and Proventil inhaler centrally stored. Prepare all doses of oral meds, crush if allowed and mix with applesauce. She can take med cup and swallow herself. **Be sure she swallows meds.** Encourage fluids. Ask about Proventil use, check container daily. First Nationwide Home Health Care client.

7 AM		Apply TAC cream to rash on forehead.
	1/2	Capoten 25 mg (=12.5 mg—already halved in bubble card)
Breakfast	1	Cephalexin 250 mg cap (until gone: should be 9/5/96)
	1	Allopurinol 300 mg
	1	TheoDur 200 mg (do not crush)
	1	furosemide 20 mg
	1	furosemide 40 mg
	1	Haldol 0.5 mg
	1	Even days only Ecotrin (in top drawer, don't crush)
	1	drop Pilocarpine 1% to her LEFT eye
	1	drop Timoptic XE to LEFT eye about 15 min. after pilocarpine
	1	Tbsp Metamucil in 6 oz of juice
9:30 AM	2	Puffs Proventil MDI (Use spacer, be sure she waits 1-2 min in between)
12 Noon	1/2	Capoten 25 mg (=12.5 mg—already halved in bubble card)
	1	drop Pilocarpine 1% in LEFT eye
	1	Cephalexin 250 mg cap (until gone; should be 9/5/96)
	1	Haldol 1 mg
		Apply TAC cream to forehead before lunch
2:30 PM	2	Puffs Proventil MDI (Use spacer, be sure she waits 1-2 min in between)
Dinner	1	Cephalexin 250 mg cap (until gone; should be 9/5/96)
	30 mL	Potassium Chloride 10% (Bottom left drawer)
	1/2	Capoten 25 mg (=12.5—already halved in bubble card)
		Apply TAC cream to forehead before dinner
9 PM	1	TheoDur 200 mg (do not crush)
	2	Puffs Proventil MDI (Use spacer, be sure she waits 1-2 min in between)
		Apply TAC cream to forehead before bed
	1	Cephalexin 250 mg cap (until gone; should be 9/5/96)

PRN meds (only at resident's request for the symptoms in the order—record all use in her record): Tylenol ES 500 mg, 2 caps every 4 hours for pain, but not more than 4 doses per day. Dulcolax suppository if no BM for 2 days. Restoril 15 mg at bedtime or after for sleep. Proventil inhaler, 2 puffs every 4 hours in-between regular use for shortness of breath.

Other Care Notes: Check on her during the night at **midnight, 2AM, 3AM, 4AM, 5AM and 6AM.** Change her sleeping position each time and make sure she is dry. Help her use her oxygen whenever she requests. Change humidifier water every even day (containers kept in cabinet under humidifier). Call daughter (Marti Gordon—445-5014) for more supplies.

low the manufacturer's recommendation on the container or package insert. It is a good idea to keep a record of the resident's use of each medication (Figure 4-2).

Therapeutic Effects and Side-Effects

There are no entirely safe medications, and while all offer desired, or therapeutic effects, each medication also has the potential to cause undesirable side-effects. The term adverse drug reaction refers to undesirable effects that may be hazardous. Side-effects may be simply an exaggeration of the intended (therapeutic) effect of the drug. That is, the dose used may cause too much of the intended effect, or the drug itself simply may be too strong for a particular resident. For example, a drug used to treat high blood pressure may cause the blood pressure to fall too low, which can result in fainting or other complications; tranquilizers or calming agents often cause sedation or drowsiness. Most side-effects, however, are not just a result of too large a dose or too sensitive a patient. For example, many drugs can cause an uncomfortable feeling or nausea because of stomach irritation. Other common side-effects, depending on the medication, are drowsiness, confusion and mental changes, headaches, dry mouth, constipation, diarrhea, fast heartbeat, insomnia, and fatigue.

There are many side-effects that can be detected, at least in the beginning, only through laboratory testing of a resident's blood. In these tests, drugs that have the potential to cause liver, blood, or kidney problems can be monitored and problems can be detected before serious harm occurs. Blood tests are also used to see if the dose a person is taking is high enough to achieve the desired effect or if it is too high. Doctors and nurses also rely on monitoring the "vital signs" of blood pressure, pulse rates, and respirations to evaluate the effectiveness of a drug and identify possible side-effects.

Our bodies adapt quickly, and side-effects often go away after a few days or weeks, so sometimes doctors tell residents to continue a new medication in spite of the side-effects. Serious side-effects such as rashes, significant discomfort, or an undesirable change in mental status should always be reported promptly to the doctor. An allergic reaction, which may cause a severe rash or life-threatening breathing difficulties is a side-effect that may require immediate emergency care. You, as the caregiver, can assist by obtaining information about all of the medications your residents take from the pharmacy, doctor, and by reading reference materials. It is important to document any known drug allergies when a resident first moves into your facility.

FIGURE 4-2 SAMPLE AS NEEDED (PRN) MEDICATION ADMINISTRATION FORM

AS NEEDED (PRN) MEDICATION ADMINISTRATION RECORD

Name: _____

Date	Time	Medication	Dose	Reason for Use and Effect of Dose	Initial
12/2/95	8 am	Tylenol #3	1	Elbow pain – effective	BEN
12/3/95	9 pm	Restoril	15 mg	Couldn't sleep – 10 pm asleep	DMF
12/6/95	8 pm	MOM	1 Tbsp	Says she is constipated	MP
12/18/95	2 pm	Robitussin DM	10 ml	Coughing, asked for cough syrup	KA

Drug Interactions

The way drugs affect each other in the body is called drug interaction. Interactions between two or more different drugs may decrease or otherwise alter the effectiveness of a drug, for example, combining a sedative with alcohol (which is viewed as a drug when considering interactions) or taking antihistamines with tranquilizers. In both cases the sedation produced may be significant; with alcohol and sedatives or tranquilizers, the effects can be fatal.

Some undesirable interactions occur simply because the two drugs are taken at the same time, for example, if an iron pill such as ferrous sulfate or a calcium supplement is taken at the same time as the antibiotic tetracycline. The calcium and iron combine with the tetracycline in such a way as to prevent some of the tetracycline from being absorbed by the body. Interactions can also occur after drugs have been absorbed in the body. These interactions usually cause one drug or the other to become either less potent or more potent. Sometimes, even when interactions occur, doctors will continue the medication, making dosage adjustments based on laboratory tests or careful observation of the resident.

Drug-food interactions usually affect the amount of drug that is absorbed. In the tetracycline example above, the calcium contained in dairy products can interact with the medicine just as will the calcium in a Tums. Therefore, taking tetracycline with milk or cheese is not a good idea. This same kind of problem can happen with certain other drug and food combinations. In most cases, absorption is most likely to be affected by how much acid is in the stomach fluid, which varies greatly according to mealtimes and amount of food in the stomach. As a general rule, drugs are more quickly and completely absorbed on an empty stomach, but there are important exceptions. Having food in the stomach helps to decrease or eliminate the most common side-effect of drugs—stomach irritation and nausea—so mealtimes are common medicine administration times as well. The resident's doctor or pharmacist should provide information whenever it is important that a particular medicine be taken before, with, or after meals. Some information on times to give medications is provided in the Medication Quick Reference.

There are also interactions with medications that are more properly called drug-diet interactions. In these cases, a person's appetite is either increased or decreased as a result of a medicine, and the outcome can be weight loss or gain. In a few cases, the drugs involved cause either a loss of taste sensation or different, unpleasant tastes, either of which can result in a loss of eating pleasure. Considering that elderly people lose some of their sense of taste and smell over time, this can be a serious problem. Some drugs, such as nasal decongestants, cause a temporary loss of appetite, and have even been sold for that purpose. A few seem to stimulate appetite and have been used for that purpose. Some antidepressants will cause weight gain on occasion, in part from decreasing the depression and the lack of appetite that often accompanies depression. Weight gain may also result from other effects of drugs that are not well understood.

It is not unusual for medications to have many potential side-effects and interactions. No one can be expected to know them all.

ALERT

Elderly persons often need a lower dose of a drug than younger persons and are more likely to have serious outcomes or side-effects. Unsteadiness caused by a drug, for example, is much more serious in an 80-year-old woman with fragile bones than in a younger person. Many falls and broken hips can be traced directly to drug side-effects. This emphasizes the importance of protecting residents by being as knowledgeable as possible about medications, including knowing what each is intended to do and at least some of the side-effects that might occur.

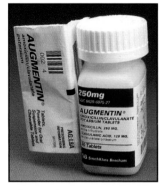

The package insert provides the same drug information that doctors refer to when prescribing medications and managing treatment.

LABELING

The labeling requirements for prescription drugs are very different from those for OTC drugs. Manufacturers of prescription drugs must include a "package insert" as part of the labeling that goes with each drug container sold to a pharmacy. These inserts are approved by the Food and Drug Administration (FDA) and contain all relevant information—the generic and chemical name of the drug, what uses it is approved for, side-effects and other cautionary statements, how it works, how it should be stored, what doses and dose forms it comes in, and how and in what doses it should be administered. These inserts are lengthy, and are not intended for laypersons.

When a prescription drug is dispensed by a pharmacy, the only labeling that is normally required is what state laws stipulate.

Common label elements are the name, address, and phone number of the pharmacy, the doctor's name, patient's name, date of dispensing, and directions for use. State laws usually require the name and strength of the drug, the quantity, and expiration date of the medication. Special instructions such as to shake liquids before use, to store the medicine in a refrigerator, or to give with food or take on an empty stomach or with large amounts of liquids are included as standard practice in many areas, although not always required by state laws. New state and federal laws also require more extensive information regarding proper administration and possible side-effects, but this is not uniformly done in all states or jurisdictions. Many pharmacies and their customers find it helpful to list the number of remaining refills on the label each time a medication is dispensed. That way, the person responsible for reordering a new supply knows to order well in advance of need so that the pharmacy can obtain the doctor's approval for new refills.

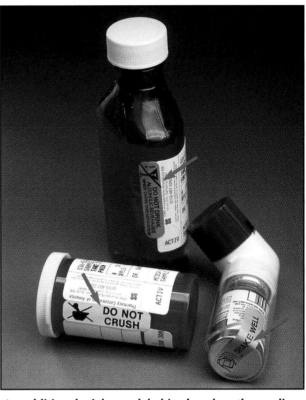

An additional sticker or label is placed on the medication at the pharmacy to alert the user to special instructions such as not to crush a particular medication or to shake the contents before use.

Labeling of OTC drugs assumes that people purchase and use these medications without consulting a doctor or pharmacist first. As a result, much of the information concerning proper storage and use, along with precautions, is included on the medication label. The generic name is always included, usually under *active ingredients*. However, just as for prescription drugs, there is often too much information to fit on the label of the container, even with the small print that is often

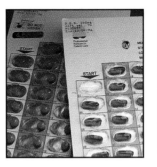

Single-dose packaging.

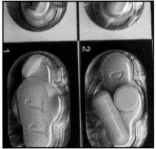

Multi-dose packaging.

used. In this case, manufacturers add a simplified package insert that includes the required information, sometimes in a box containing the medicine bottle, sometimes affixed to the bottle by glue or plastic wrapping. These inserts contain useful information and should be kept with the container whenever possible.

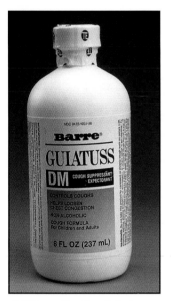

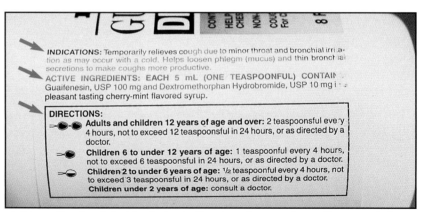

INDICATIONS: Temporarily relieves cough due to minor throat and bronchial irritation as may occur with a cold. Helps loosen phlegm (mucus) and thin bronchial
secretions to make coughs more productive.
ACTIVE INGREDIENTS: EACH 5 mL (ONE TEASPOONFUL) CONTAINS
Guaifenesin, USP 100 mg and Dextromethorphan Hydrobromide, USP 10 mg in a
pleasant tasting cherry-mint flavored syrup.

DIRECTIONS:
Adults and children 12 years of age and over: 2 teaspoonsful every
4 hours, not to exceed 12 teaspoonsful in 24 hours, or as directed by a
doctor.
Children 6 to under 12 years of age: 1 teaspoonful every 4 hours,
not to exceed 6 teaspoonsful in 24 hours, or as directed by a doctor.
Children 2 to under 6 years of age: ½ teaspoonful every 4 hours, not
to exceed 3 teaspoonsful in 24 hours, or as directed by a doctor.
Children under 2 years of age: consult a doctor.

OTC medication label includes indications for use, ingredients, and dos-
ing instructions.

OTC medication labels
show the drug name and
actions and the expected
benefits.

WARNINGS: Do not take this product for persistent or chronic cough such as occurs w
smoking, asthma, chronic bronchitis, or emphysema, or where cough is accompanied
excessive phlegm (mucus) unless directed by a doctor. A persistent cough may be a sig
a serious condition. If cough persists for more than 1 week, tends to recur, or is accom
ied by a fever, rash, or persistent headache, consult a doctor. As with any drug, if you
pregnant or nursing a baby, seek the advice of a health professional before using this p
ct. Keep this and all drugs out of the reach of children. In case of accidental overd
eek professional assistance or contact a poison control center immediately.
Drug Interaction Precaution: Do not use this product if you are now taking a prescrip
monoamine oxidase inhibitor (MAOI) (certain drugs for depression, psychiatric or e
ional conditions, or Parkinson's disease), or for 2 weeks after stopping the MAOI dru
you are uncertain whether your prescription drug contains an MAOI, consult a he
professional before taking this product.
DO NOT ACCEPT IF CAP SEAL IMPRINTED WITH ⓣ IS BROKEN OR MISSING

OTC medication label includes warnings, precautions, drug interactions,
and special instructions.

In most pharmacies, prescription drugs in tablet or capsule form are usually packaged in one of two ways—in the manufacturer's original container, with the pharmacy label applied on top of the manufacturer's, or repackaged in plastic vials. Residential care facilities that assume responsibility for centralized storage and assistance with administration can obtain these medications in cards with foil backing and individual doses in plastic bubbles. These are called "punch cards," "bubble cards," "bingo cards," and sometimes even "unit dose" packages.

Federal law requires that all drugs be in containers that have closures (caps, lids) that are "child resistant." However, many elderly persons with poor eyesight or arthritis have found this packaging to be equally "elderly resistant." As a result, laws have been changed to allow persons to request and obtain prescription and OTC drugs with regular caps or lids.

Guidelines and Techniques

Doctor's Orders

How can you ensure that your residents who need assistance with medications take their medications properly? The first step is to be sure you know how the resident's doctor wants the medications to be taken. Most caregivers rely on the prescription label but, when pharmacies have been given authority to refill prescriptions in advance, they do not check with doctors to see if the directions are still current. If the doctor tells the resident to change directions for use from, for example, two tablets a day to three, the pharmacy will not know and the prescription label will be wrong. The best way to prevent this is to ask the doctor to give you or the resident instructions in writing when directions are changed. Some doctors will write a new prescription, which should be sent to the dispensing pharmacy after noting the information in a resident's record or on a medication administration record or other medication scheduling form (Figure 4-1). Most state laws do not permit relabeling of medications by caregivers, but a "direction change" sticker or other simple notation on the container will remind you to tell the pharmacy of any changes so the pharmacist will know to check with the doctor before refilling the prescription.

Another method is to send the doctor a copy of the current medication "orders" each time a resident visits the doctor. The doctor can then make any changes directly on the record and return it to the facility. If a new medication is prescribed, be sure it is ordered from the pharmacy, either by the doctor directly or by written prescription taken or faxed to the pharmacy.

Scheduling

Instructions for taking medications are usually given in one of two ways. The first is based on a certain number of times each day, sometimes specifying what time of day to take them. These are often referred to as "routine" medications. The second includes medicines ordered "as needed" (PRN), usually with some sort of limit, such as "every 4 hours." Caregivers are usually able to assist with routine drugs without much problem. The important issues to consider are:

- Make certain you know the current directions for use.
- Help your resident follow directions correctly.
- Be certain the proper dose is prepared and taken.

• Stay alert for possible problems resulting from the use of the medications.

These issues are discussed in more detail later in this section. It is also important to understand the need to follow the doctor's orders as closely as possible, for both PRN and routine drugs.

Routine medication orders for more than one dose per day should be spread out evenly through waking hours. Doctors will usually specify a certain spacing or state "around the clock" when it is necessary to take the medication during the night—for example, give every 8 hours. Figure 4-3 is one example of a prescription medication record that will help document a resident's adherence to prescribed therapy.

PRN medications present a different challenge, because most states do not allow caregivers to make determinations of need. However, most do allow assistance with administration once the resident asks for a particular PRN drug based on his or her own perception of need. Caregivers are usually permitted to offer PRN medications when the need is apparent ("Would you like your Robitussin for that cough?"). In these cases caregiver responsibilities are primarily to ensure that the limits of the order (such as, "every 4 hours if needed for pain") or, in the case of OTC drugs, the manufacturer's recommendations, are not exceeded if the caregiver has assumed responsibility for control of the resident's medications. It is also advisable to keep a record of PRN use (see Figure 4-2) and the resident's response to the medication, especially when there appears to be a sharp increase over previous use. This may help to determine if the resident's doctor needs to be contacted.

Additional information you can obtain from the pharmacist includes:

• Which medications must be refrigerated or stored in a cool place

• When a liquid must be shaken well before use

• When the medication expires

• When to take a medication with large amounts of liquid

• What foods or other medications not to take with a particular medicine

• Whether to take before, with, or after meals

FIGURE 4-3 SAMPLE MEDICATION RECORD FORM

MEDICATIONS	HOUR	1	2	3	4	5	6	7	8	9	10	11	12	13	14	15	16	17	18	19	20	21	22	23	24	25	26	27	28	29	30	31
1. Digoxin 0.125 mg QD	8	✔	✔																													
2. Keflex 250 mg QID	8	✔	✔																													
	12	✔	✔																													
	4	R	R																													
	8	R	R																													
3. Tylenol #3 Q4H PRN pain																																
4. Robitussin DM 10 cc Q4H PRN cough																																
5.																																
6.																																
7.																																
8.																																
9.																																
10.		1	2	3	4	5	6	7	8	9	10	11	12	13	14	15	16	17	18	19	20	21	22	23	24	25	26	27	28	29	30	31

ALLERGIES: Sulfa   SPECIAL INSTRUCTIONS: Needs help with all meds

PHYSICIAN: PHONE: FACILITY

NAME   #   ROOM/BED NUMBER: SEX: D.O.B.   /   /   DATE:

2-8-82-110	**MEDICATION RECORD**				A.M.								P.M.								◯
		1	2	3	4	5	6	7	8	9	10	11	12	1	2	3	4	5	6	7	8	9	10	11	12

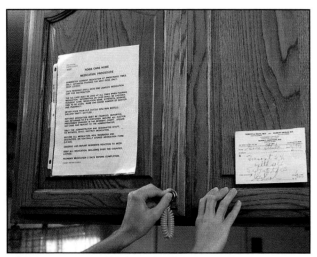

Locked, centrally located medication cabinet.

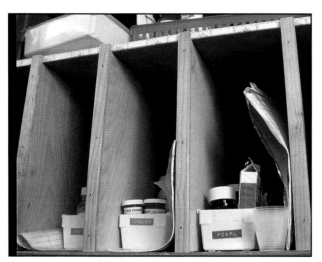

Separation and labeling of each resident's medications.

Storage

Proper storage is an important part of assisting residents. For example, if medications are not kept in a secure place other residents could take them inadvertently and suffer considerable harm. If medications are not stored under proper temperature, light, and moisture controls, they can lose their effectiveness, especially if stored improperly for a long time. Proper storage also means providing a well-lighted area and enough separation between different residents' medicines to help prevent errors by the caregiver. Refrigerators containing medicines should be kept between 36 and 46 degrees Fahrenheit; temperature can be monitored with a thermometer. Room temperatures over 86 degrees Fahrenheit for hours at a time can alter the effectiveness of some drugs.

Preparing Medications

The actual preparation of doses to be taken by residents should take into consideration the degree of assistance needed, the dose schedule, and caregiver availability for the task. The following steps are recommended, but remember to check with state agencies if you have any question about your legal responsibility.

- Use a medication schedule for each resident who needs assistance of any kind, including those who just need reminders to take the medications they store in their rooms.

- Try to prepare doses away from distractions, in an area with good lighting.

- Use mealtimes when possible to establish a consistent, reliable time for residents to take medications. Be sure your schedule identifies medications that should be taken on an empty stomach (45 minutes to an hour before meals or at least 2 hours after meals in most cases).

- When you store medications centrally, but the resident will actually take the dose from the container, remove those containers from storage and set aside. Be sure that the directions for use on the label are correct and that you have something you can check when the resident takes his or her own medications.

- When you are going to prepare the actual doses for administration, it is recommended that you put medications in a container, such as a paper cup labeled with the resident's name, instead of placing medications on a

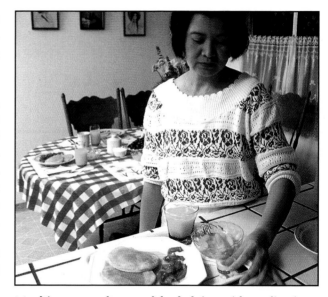

Mealtimes are often used for helping with medications.

plate or other object at the table. It is important to give medications to each person individually and wait to be sure the medications are swallowed.

- Take measures to ensure the privacy of residents administering eye drops, nose drops, or sprays, and medications given by routes other than by mouth. Some residents may object to taking even oral medicines in front of others, and that feeling must be respected.

- Be sure there is plenty of water or other liquid available when residents are taking medications. Many older persons fail to drink enough fluids during the day, and this is a good time to encourage more fluid intake. Most water glasses and coffee mugs hold a cup (8 oz.) of fluid. Teacups average about 6 oz. of fluid.

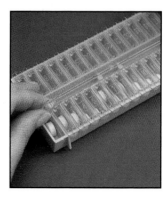

Daily medication counter.

- Even though residents may place their own medications into different containers, such as a pill box or daily-dose reminder, preparing an entire day's medication doses at once for later use can be hazardous and is *illegal* for caregivers to do in many states. There are systems available from some pharmacies that package all the oral pills for a given dosage time together in separate plastic "bubbles" as part of a "punch card" system. The disadvantage is the possibility that changes ordered by the doctor will not be made. There is also a slight possibility that 2 uncoated tablets stored together would not be chemically compatible over time.

- Although not usually required by state regulations, it can be helpful to keep track of when residents choose not to take medication doses as ordered. A person has the right to choose not to comply with prescribed therapy, but this can result in more serious health problems. Informing the doctor that a resident frequently refuses routine medication will help him or her determine what adjustments in therapy are needed. For example, if the doctor does not know that a resident has refused to take seizure medication just prior to giving a blood sample to determine the amount of that drug in the body, the doctor may adjust the dose higher than it should be, resulting in possible side-effects or toxicity when the resident takes the medication according to the new directions for use.

- Most medications in liquid form allow for some error in measuring. However, household teaspoons have measured from 3.5 ml (milliliters) to 7 ml (the standard is 5 ml). Whenever possible, it is preferable to use specially designed and calibrated medication "spoons" or cups for accurate measurement. Be sure to rinse out any measuring device that is not disposable, and only reuse supplies for the same resident and the same medication if they are washed in a dishwasher.

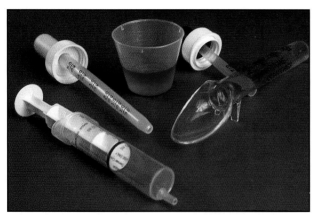

A variety of devices are available for measuring and giving oral, liquid medications.

- Use an accurate measuring "spoon" (actually a see-through plastic tube with measuring lines and a spoon-like appearance at the open end).

- Use oral dosing syringes.

- Be sure to put medication containers away promptly to ensure that a confused resident does not have access to them.

- Careful handwashing at appropriate times is always important in caring for residents to help prevent the spread of germs and reduce the potential for illness among your residents and staff. Handwashing is especially important when you will be handling medications and foods and beverages and when you or a staff person uses the bathroom or assists a resident with toileting. Specific steps are illustrated in Figure 4-4. You should include handwashing as a topic in your staff orientation and training.

FIGURE 4-4 **Handwashing**

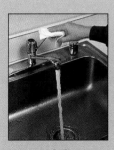 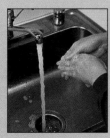 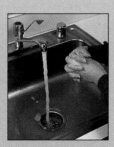 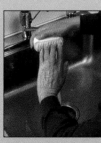 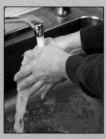

a. Avoid direct contact with bathroom surfaces by using a clean, dry paper towel to handle the water faucets.

b. Using a germicidal soap, scrub with your fingertips pointing down toward the sink drain.

c. Interlace your fingers and clean the entire surface of your hands, fingers, and wrists.

d. Use a fingernail brush or orange stick to clean beneath your fingernails.

e. Rinse your hands thoroughly, keeping your fingertips pointed down toward the drain, and use a clean, dry paper towel to turn off the faucet.

Steps to Take to Provide Medication Assistance

1. Learn medication measuring systems and terminology.
2. Identify regulations in your state regarding assistance with administration of medications.
3. Establish a system to keep track of how doctors want residents to take medications.
4. Establish a scheduling method and routine administration times.
5. Analyze resident needs including physical limitations and mental impairment.
6. Maintain proper storage areas for residents and facility.
7. Write detailed policies and procedures for medications and follow them.
8. Consider use of a fax machine for communications with doctors and pharmacists.
9. Establish a working relationship with one or more pharmacies.
10. Frequently patronize pharmacies that provide information and other services you need.
11. Ask a pharmacist to visit occasionally and consult with you and residents.
12. Set up a uniform reordering system when several pharmacies must be used.
13. Consider asking for modified packaging to improve accuracy in administration of medications.

Routes of Administration

Oral Medications

The term *pill* refers to almost any solid dosage form taken by mouth.

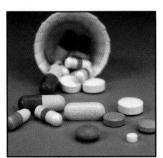

Many oral medications are prepared in a variety of tablet and capsule forms.

Tablets can be coated or uncoated. Uncoated tablets are usually white with a powdery texture. They can be chewed or swallowed whole, or can usually be easily broken. Because they absorb water easily, they dissolve fairly quickly in the stomach, although they are more likely to "stick" while swallowing, especially if taken without adequate fluids.

The person chewing or swallowing the tablet can usually taste the medication, so very bitter or bad-tasting medicines in tablet form are often given a thin, hard-shell coating. This coating sometimes causes problems when people try to break a tablet in half; some tablets shatter into smaller pieces.

Some tablets are scored; that is, a small groove is made in a line across the tablet to allow it to be broken accurately into two halves without having to cut it. Many people with arthritis find it difficult to break tablets in half, even if scored. Some pharmacies will break the tablets for residents, but there are also gadgets available in pharmacies to help. The simplest kind is a small plastic-hinged device that contains a razor-type implement (see Figure 4-5). The result is almost always a clean break with equal halves. Kitchen knives, razor blades, etc., can also be used.

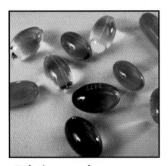

Gelatin capsules.

Extended or long-acting tablets, covered under "Sustained-Release Medications," should not be cut or broken unless the manufacturer specifically permits it (your pharmacist will know when that is the case).

Capsules will either be in hard gelatin shells containing powders that usually can be pulled apart or in single soft gelatin pods that contain a syrupy liquid. These cannot be pulled apart, but can be punctured and the liquid squeezed out. Do not try to adjust dosage by removing part of the powder or liquid in capsules; that could be unsafe. Capsules dissolve quickly in the stomach, are usually easy to swallow, and cause no taste problems. If capsules are emptied into food or a liquid, be sure to empty the capsule completely.

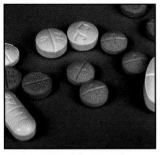

A scored tablet can be split into two equal halves.

Troches, lozenges, and similar products are designed to dissolve slowly in the mouth, usually to provide a topical effect in the mouth or throat. Medications in this dosage form may include anything from cough suppressants to hard candy. To reduce the pos-

Figure 4-5 **Splitting a Tablet**

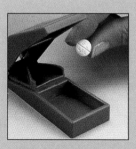

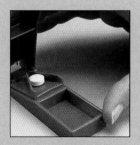

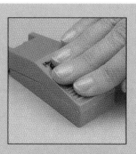

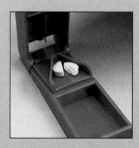

a. The tablet is most likely to split properly if it is scored.

b. Place the tablet on the bottom platform.

c. Close the lid containing the razor blade over the tablet.

d. Check to be certain the tablet has been split evenly.

sibility of choking it is important that residents who take these medicines have no difficulty swallowing.

Liquid medications are especially useful for persons who have difficulty swallowing tablets or capsules, for those with nasal gastric or gastrostomy tubes, and for medication doses not available in tablet form in the dose the doctor wants to use. Because the drug is already dissolved or in very small particles, liquid forms are also often easier on the stomach than tablets or capsules.

Syrups are sweet-flavored liquids that contain medications in a dissolved form. They can usually be diluted with water if necessary just before taking. Shaking before use is not usually needed, but a quick shake or two before pouring out a dose is probably a good idea. Many cough and cold medications are in syrup form.

Suspensions are liquid dose forms that contain medicine in suspended form, not dissolved, so it is very important to shake the bottle well (8 to 10 times). Otherwise, the resident can get too little or too much medication. Suspensions can usually be diluted with water if needed, but only just before administration and only with an amount approved by the pharmacist or doctor. Examples of suspensions you are likely to see include milk of magnesia and phenytoin (Dilantin) suspension.

"Elixirs," "solutions," and "liquids" are medicines in a flavored liquid. Sometimes the liquid is part alcohol. Some mixing with water is usually OK, but if the liquid has a fairly high alcohol content, that can result in the medication falling out of solution, and you will actually see the medication (as particles that float or settle to the bottom) in the liquid. Always check with the pharmacist or doctor regarding the dilution of medications. Improper dilution could lead to problems in administration and even in the effectiveness of the drug.

Effervescent tablets become solutions or suspensions after water is added. They should be stirred, not shaken, and the tablets should not be crushed or chewed.

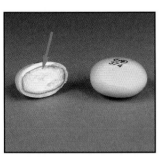

A time-release medication should not be split. This tablet is manufactured with an inner core, which dissolves later than the outer portion of the tablet.

Sustained- and Delayed-Release Medications have many advantages. Sustained-release preparations ensure that the medication will be released evenly over a period of time (8 to 24 hours, depending on the product). This maintains levels of the drug in the body. Enteric-coated tablets or capsules only delay release of the medicine until after the tablet is past the stomach. Enteric coatings protect some drugs against breakdown by stomach acids, and protect the stomach against the irritation caused by other medications.

Sustained- or delayed-release tablets and capsules should never be crushed or chewed. Capsules can be opened and mixed with foods like applesauce, or they can be added to liquids just before taking. Some sustained-release tablets can be broken into smaller pieces to make swallowing easier. Always check with the pharmacy before breaking any sustained-release tablet, unless the directions for use clearly specify that it is OK to do so.

Even though sustained-release medications are only going to be taken once or twice a day, it is still very important to be sure that they are administered at the correct times.

Medication Identification. All prescription drug tablets and capsules are manufactured with an identifying number or mark. This enables poison control centers and others to quickly identify the drug name and strength. Many brand name pills are now marked with the name of the drug and/or manufacturer as well as the strength of the drug.

Crushing Tablets. When uncoated tablets must be crushed to make it easier for the resident to swallow, it is not usually necessary to crush them very fine. Using a spoon and another hard surface such as a cup or saucer (being careful not to scatter pieces of the tablet in the process) will work in most cases. There are also special devices used in health facilities that work quickly and effectively for this purpose. These devices can also be used to crush the hard-coated shells (not the delayed-release shell) of some tablets. Mortars and pestles are also very effective (see Figure 4-6). It is a good idea, when-

FIGURE 4-6 **Crushing a Tablet**

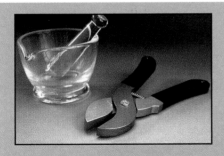

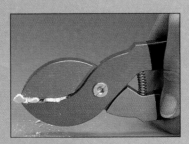
Mortar and pestle and pill-crushing device.

Mortar and Pestle

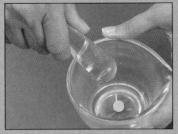
a. Place tablet in the bottom of the mortar.

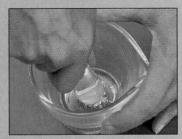
b. Use the pestle to grind the tablet.

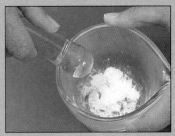
c. Check to be certain tablet is properly crushed.

Pill Crusher

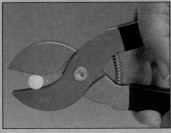
a. Put pill into pill crusher.

b. Crush pill.

ever possible, to use two paper "soufflé" cups when crushing tablets. Place the tablet or tablets in one, then place the second cup on top of the pills inside the first cup, and crush the tablets between the two cups. Make sure all medication powder is scraped off the bottom of the top cup into the bottom cup. If crushing directly with a mortar and pestle or special device, be sure to empty out the entire dose and clean the device before crushing another resident's medications. Even very small amounts of residue can cause an allergic reaction in another resident.

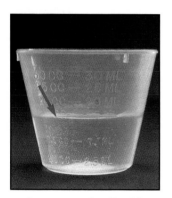

When measuring liquid medications, hold the container at eye level and measure to the meniscus line—the level of liquid at the center of the container.

If a resident has problems swallowing pills, ask the doctor if the same medicine is available in liquid form from the pharmacy.

Measuring Liquids. An example of a measuring device you can obtain at the pharmacy or from your wholesale suppliers is a transparent plastic medicine cup. These are convenient, inexpensive, and easy to use, and can be used to measure a wide variety of doses with reasonable accuracy. When using these cups, they should be held up to eye level and the dose line embossed on the cup lined up with the "meniscus line," which is the lower portion of the curved line at the top of the liquid in the cup.

You should note that most liquid dose forms are not so potent that a small variation in dose will make very much of a difference to your resident. It is important, however, to start with measuring equipment that is as accurate as possible; then small errors in measuring technique will not become significant errors in dosage. Potent drugs in liquid form usually come with a calibrated dropper that allows for very accurate measurement.

In most cases, liquids can and should be taken with water or juice. This helps to reduce the bad taste of some liquids. There are a few instances in which a particular liquid will not mix well with liquids other than water. As a general rule, it is better to mix the medication with clear liquids such as juices or punch instead of milk or other liquids that are cloudy or opaque. Ask your pharmacist if you have any doubts. Sometimes liquids with a disagreeable taste can be given cold to minimize the bad taste.

Sublingual Medications (Figure 4-7a) are placed under the tongue, where they quickly dissolve and are quickly absorbed into the many blood vessels present there. Sublingual medications produce a quicker response than is possible when they must first pass through the stomach. Nitroglycerin is the drug most often given sublingually.

Buccal Medication administration (Figure 4-7b) involves placing the medication inside the mouth between the cheek pouches and the gums, which also have many blood vessels close to the surface. Buccal administration offers the same advantages as sublingual administration.

Medications Applied to the Skin for Systemic Use

One of the more recent developments in medicine is the transdermal (through the skin) drug delivery system (see Figure 4-8). This system uses skin patches that release medicine slowly and steadily for periods ranging from 24 hours to 7 days. These are usually called "patches" and they are especially valuable when people forget when to take their medications or when periodic dosing is ineffective.

FIGURE 4-7 **Sublingual and Buccal Administration**

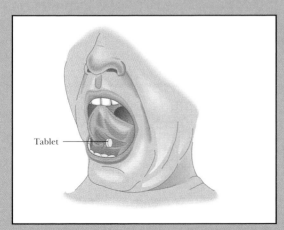

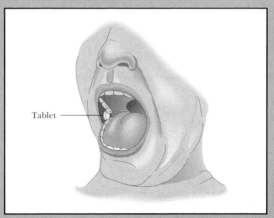

a. Sublingual medications are placed under the tongue.

b. Buccal administration involves placing the medication between the cheek and gum.

FIGURE 4-8 **Transdermal Drug Delivery System**

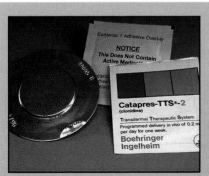

Medicated skin patch.

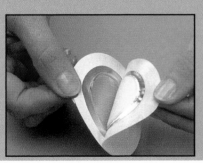

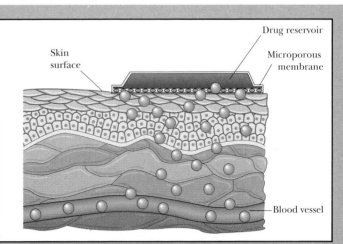

This transdermal patch delivers medication into the bloodstream in a consistent, controlled manner.

Be certain that the medicated patch, not the adhesive backing, is applied to the skin.

When applying patches, it is important to remove the old patch first and to rotate the locations so that the patches will not cause irritation to the skin. Most patches hold securely, but it is a good idea to check each day to be sure a patch has not fallen off after bathing or been accidentally removed in one's sleep. Never apply a patch without being sure that the previous one is removed first. Although the patches may look harmless, they contain powerful drugs.

Also be sure that the medicated side of the patch is applied to the skin. Even licensed nurses have applied the protective cover that comes with some patches instead of the patch itself.

The most common patches in current use are Nitroglycerin patches for angina or chest pain, Catapres patches for high blood pressure, Scopolamine patches for motion sickness, nicotine patches for people who are trying to quit smoking, and Duragesic (a narcotic for pain relief).

Eye Drops and Ointments

These preparations are referred to as "ophthalmics." They are applied directly to or around the eye, sometimes to treat long-standing conditions such as glaucoma, sometimes to cure infections or treat irritations, and, especially in the elderly, to help lubricate dry eyes (see Figures 4-9a and 4-9b).

Eye preparations are sterile and usually contain a preservative to keep germs from growing in them because the eye is very susceptible to infection. For this reason, it is important to have clean hands when administering eye drops or ointments, to keep the applicator tip clean by not touching anything with it, including the eye, and by keeping it tightly closed when not using it. As a general rule, even though eye drops contain preservatives, it is a good idea to discard them after they have been open for 6 months or so, even if the expiration date has not passed.

When residents have more than one eye drop to administer at the same time, they should wait at least 5 minutes between different preparations to allow the first drop to be absorbed. Occasionally, it is necessary to wait at least 10 minutes. Eye ointments should be administered after eye drops, if both are ordered. Administration of eye medicines requires careful attention and an ability to manipulate a very small container close to a resident's eye. For this reason, some people with arthritis or tremors cannot administer their own eye drops.

Most eye medications fall under one of the following categories:

1. Antibiotics for eye infections. These drops may be in the form of suspensions that should be moderately or lightly shaken before use, or they may be in ointment form.

2. Cortisone products for irritations or allergies that result in reddened, painful, or itching eyes.

3. Eye drops for glaucoma must be used very carefully; often one eye requires a different strength of the medicine than the other eye. These medicines will be needed for life. Many persons with glaucoma must use more than one eye medication.

4. Artificial tears to help when the eyes do not produce enough tears to adequately lubricate the eye. "Dry eyes" are itchy and uncomfortable and common in the elderly. Artificial tears should not be used at the same time as other eye medications. Artificial tears do not require a prescription and are used by many elderly persons for the rest of their lives.

5. Eye washes can be useful for washing small particles of debris from the eye and are refreshing to many people. They are available OTC.

ALERT

Read eye drop labels very carefully because printing is usually very small and most containers and even some labels look almost identical. Eye drops and ear drops often are dispensed in very similar containers. Use of ear drops in the eye may cause severe irritation.

Never use one person's eye medication for another person.

Techniques for the Administration of Eye Medications

Step 1: Wash hands thoroughly and dry with a clean towel. Latex gloves may also be used.

Step 2: Position the resident with his or her head tilted back and the eye open.

FIGURE 4-9a **Eye Drops**

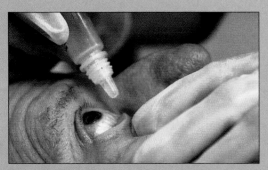

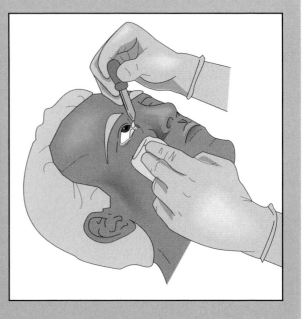

Gently retract the lower portion of the eye-lid away from the eye so that it forms a pouch. Carefully squeeze the dropper to place the medication into the eyelid pouch.

FIGURE 4-9b **Eye Ointments**

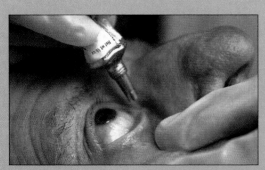

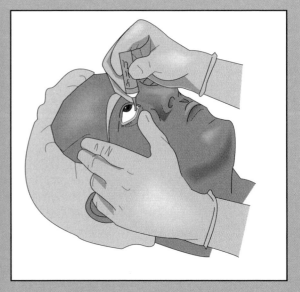

Gently retract the lower portion of the eye-lid away from the eye so that it forms a pouch. Gently squeeze about 1/3 inch of ointment into and across the pouch.

Step 3: Remove the cap from the eye drop container and place it carefully on a clean, dry surface or hold it between two fingers on one hand.

Step 4: Using your other hand, gently retract the lower portion of the eyelid away from the eye so that it forms a pouch.

Step 5: Carefully squeeze the dropper to place the medication into the eyelid pouch. Be careful not to touch any part of the eye with the dropper. For ointments, gently squeeze about 1/3 inch into and across the pouch.

Step 6: Gently close the eye and keep it closed for a minute or two. In some cases, the resident may be instructed to *gently* rub across the eye to help evenly distribute the medication; in other cases the instructions may be to put *light* pressure against the corner of the eye for a few moments after instilling the drop. Be sure you know *how* the doctor wants the drops instilled. If a second drop is ordered, instill after 2 or 3 minutes. If another ophthalmic medication is to be instilled in the same eye, wait at least 5 minutes before instilling the second one.

Step 7: Wash your hands again.

If the pharmacy only labels the box that an eye preparation comes in, be sure to save it, and always return the bottle or tube to its original container. In most cases, ophthalmic products can be stored at controlled room temperature (up to 86 degrees Fahrenheit). Only a very few must be refrigerated.

Ear Medications

Ear medications or otics are those that are dropped into the ear canal, rather than on the outside surface of the ear. Ear medications are of two basic types: those that aid in the removal of wax or fluids and those that are used to treat infections in the ear. Sometimes wax-removal medications are used in conjunction with a special ear syringe, which can be used to help remove fluids or dissolved wax or to irrigate the ear. Never use a container of ear drops for more than one resident, and do not reuse ear syringes without first thoroughly sanitizing them (see Figure 4-10).

The ear is not as likely to become infected as the eye, but cleanliness is nevertheless important in the administration process. The main concern is to keep the drops from running out of the ear until they have been given time to penetrate the infection site or the hardened wax, and then to leave them there long enough to do some good. This usually means having the resident lie with his or her head turned to one side for a period of time. When removing ear wax, warming the ear drop bottle in a container of warm water or by holding it in your closed hand for a few minutes is almost always useful. Sometimes residents will be told to plug the ear with cotton after filling the ear canal to keep the medicine there longer while still allowing for movement. This makes it easier to retain the medication, but the plug itself will absorb much of the medicine and draw it out from the ear canal.

FIGURE 4-10 **Ear Drops**

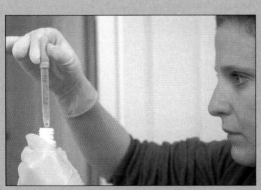
Draw prescribed amount into dropper.

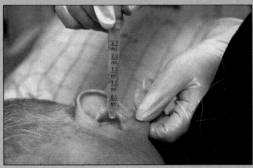
Pull ear lobe down and back and drop the required dose into the ear canal.

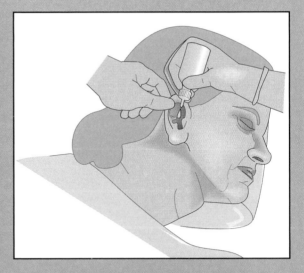

Techniques for the Administration of Ear Drops

Step 1: Wash hands.

Step 2: Have resident lie down with affected ear up or tilt head to one side with the affected ear up.

Step 3: Gently pull the ear lobe downward and backward (this straightens the ear canal).

Step 4: Drop the required dose into the ear canal. Try not to touch the tip of the dropper to anything, and replace the lid or the dropper promptly. If the tip touched anything, or there is medication around the tip, wipe it off with a clean paper towel or tissue before replacing.

Step 5: Have the resident maintain the same position for 5 to 10 minutes to allow the medication to penetrate the target area. It may be necessary to gently plug the ear with cotton (sterile is preferred, especially if the ear is infected) to prevent excessive leakage.

Nasal (Nose) Preparations

Most nose drops and sprays are used to relieve nasal or sinus congestion, and are available OTC. A small number of medications are administered for their systemic effect (throughout the body) or for effect lower in the respiratory tract. These medications require a prescription. Follow directions supplied by the doctor carefully, and check with the doctor or pharmacist if there are questions about how to administer these medications. Be sure the nasal passage is clear before administering nose drops or sprays.

Nasal decongestants can cause a more serious congestion known as "rebound" congestion if overused. It is important to use decongestants only as recommended. Non-medicated salt-solution (saline) nose drops are often used to simply clear the nose and are less expensive than decongestants (see Figure 4-11).

FIGURE 4-11 **Nose Drops**

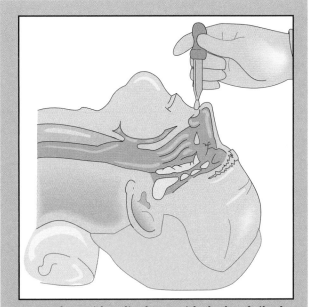

Have the resident lie down with the head tilted back and carefully squeeze a few drops into one or both notstrils.

Techniques for the Administration of Nasal Spray

Step 1: Wash hands.

Step 2: Have resident gently blow nose.

Step 3: *For drops:* Have the resident lie down on his or her back with the head tilted over the back of a pillow or over the side of a bed. Carefully squeeze a few drops into one or both nostrils.

  For spray: Hold head erect and spray quickly and forcefully 2 or 3 times while the resident "sniffs" quickly and forcefully. Although the force applied to nasal spray containers is intended to penetrate far enough up the nose to reach the swollen vessels, gravity is a big help, and spray can be as effective as drops if the head is tilted back when spray is used.

Step 4: Wait a minute or two, then blow nose gently again. Repeat the process once if the treatment was not effective.

Step 5: Wipe the dropper or sprayer with a tissue, then rinse in hot water (keep it pointed downward so water does not get into it) and replace the cap.

Step 6: Wash hands again.

Vaporizers and Humidifiers

Cool mist vaporizers and steam humidifiers have been used for many years to help with breathing problems and nasal and bronchial congestion. They can help to make breathing easier by adding cool mist to the air, but have no medicinal value.

Multiple-Dose or Metered-Dose Inhalers

Multiple-dose or metered-dose inhalers (MDIs) come in small metal canisters and deliver a measured dose under pressure each time the stem valve is depressed. Some of the medications in these containers are also available with hand-held nebulizers, devices that provide essentially the same small droplets of medication to the patient's airways. Nebulizers can be more effective than inhalers, but only if the person using them is skilled in their use (see Figure 4-12).

  Overuse of these medications can result in decreased effectiveness. This is particularly true of the ones that are available over-the-counter. Because people with breathing difficulties sometimes become very anxious about their condition, there is always a concern about overuse.

FIGURE 4-12 **Inhalers**

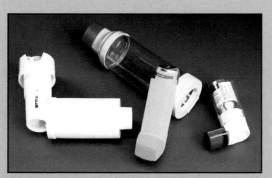

Multiple- or Metered-Dose Inhalers.

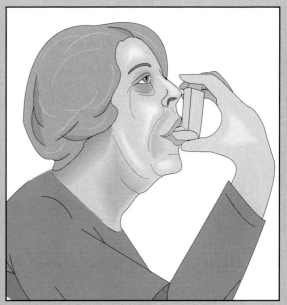

Technique for the use of an inhaler.

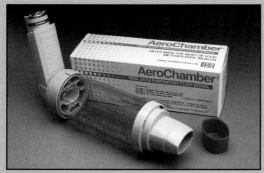

Spacer fitted with metered-dose inhaler.

There are currently four different types of inhalers used in chronic obstructive pulmonary disease (COPD), asthma, and other respiratory conditions. These inhalers dilate the bronchial tubes, making breathing easier. Often, doctors will prescribe three different solutions, to be used one after the other, up to 4 or more times a day. One of the medications is a drug that immediately opens the airways. Examples include albuterol (Proventil, Ventolin, Alupent, Brethine) and several OTC products containing epinephrine (Adrenalin, Primatene Mist, Bronkaid). Another medication, Ipratropium (Atrovent), works in a different way, but is also fast-acting. The third type of MDI contains a cortisone-like drug. This drug is used last if administered with other MDIs, and the mouth should be rinsed with water after use (do not swallow the water) to prevent mouth infections. Examples include beclomethasone (Beclovent, Vanceril), triamcinolone (Azmacort), and flurisolide (AeroBid). An example of the fourth type of MDI is cromolyn (Intal), which is not used as often in elderly persons. Cromolyn does not dilate the bronchial tubes; it is used primarily in asthmatic conditions.

As important as the medicine in the inhaler is the proper method of administration. Although each package includes instructions on the proper use of inhalers, everyone using these devices should be taught the proper method of administration by a nurse, doctor, pharmacist, respiratory therapist, or someone else skilled in their use. Failure to inhale deeply enough or at the proper time can prevent the medication from working properly. "Spacers" are assistive devices that help to concentrate the mist for better absorption, but even these are without much value if poor technique is used.

When more than one dose or "puff" is administered, there should be a wait of at least 1 minute (more for some) between puffs and at least 5 minutes between different kinds of medications. Be sure to read the package insert and container label. Call the resident's doctor or pharmacist if there are any questions.

Rectal Medications

Rectal medications are usually used to relieve local discomfort (hemorrhoids, local irritation, or itching), to stimulate a bowel movement, or to provide medications for nausea and pain to residents who are unable to take medications by mouth (Figure 4-13).

Techniques for the Administration of Rectal Suppositories

Step 1:   Wash your hands and put on latex gloves.

Step 2:   Apply a small amount of lubricant such as mineral oil, K-Y lubricating jelly, or petroleum jelly onto the suppository.

If the suppository was stored in a refrigerator prior to use, it is usually best to let it warm up before use. If the suppository is too soft, firm it up by holding it briefly under cold water.

Step 3:   Remove the foil or wrapping and carefully insert the suppository well past the rectal sphincter muscle. It is usually most comfortable for the person to be lying on his or her left side with the top or both knees drawn up.

Step 4:   After administration, discard gloves and wash hands again.

FIGURE 4-13 **Rectal Medications**

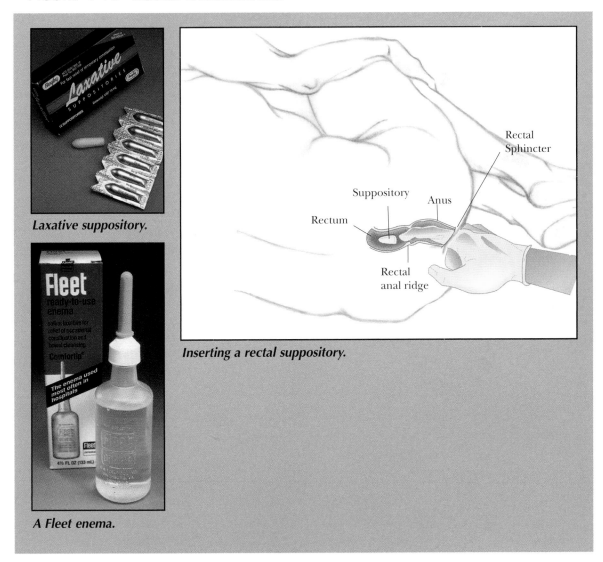

Laxative suppository.

A Fleet enema.

Inserting a rectal suppository.

Packaged rectal enemas such as Fleets, can be administered in the same position as suppositories or as outlined on the package. Remember to lubricate the tip before use, and to wash hands before and after use. Expect and be prepared for a prompt effect from an enema.

When applying other medications to the rectal area, wash hands, use gloves, and gently bathe and dry the area. Apply the medication in small amounts and rub in gently to the entire affected area. If you are using a cream or ointment that has a rectal applicator, position the resident in a similar manner to that used for administration of rectal suppositories, lubricate the applicator, and squeeze the tube gently to apply the medication. Wash the applicator thoroughly in hot soapy water, dry (or air dry), and replace on the tube. Remember to wash hands thoroughly after all procedures and to dispose of gloves quickly and properly. Never reuse a glove.

FIGURE 4-14 **Vaginal Suppository**

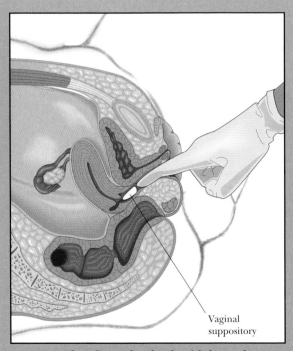

Vaginal
suppository

Have resident lie on her back with knees bent. Unwrap the suppository. Apply a small amount of lubricant onto the suppository and gently insert into the vagina.

Vaginal Medications

Vaginal medications are usually intended for local effect to treat infections or to apply estrogen to the wall of the vagina. These medications come as douches, jellies, creams, suppositories, and tablets (see Figure 4-14). Creams can be applied either locally to the vaginal area or inserted into the vagina with special applicators. Most are available by prescription only, but there are now many effective products available without a prescription for the treatment of fungal infections.

Caregivers should wash their hands before and after, wear disposable gloves, and wash reusable applicators in hot soapy water after use. Both prescription and OTC products normally give very clear instructions and diagrams for proper use, and those should be followed carefully.

Other Topical (On the Skin) Products

There are many ointments, creams, lotions, foams, sprays, powders, and solutions that contain medications intended for use on an area of the skin. Ointments are usually oil-based and act as water barriers, whereas creams are more likely to mix with water and are less noticeable on the skin. These medications are used to prevent or treat a variety of topical infections and to relieve itching, rashes, and other skin conditions. In most cases, residents will be able to apply their own ointments or creams, but some assistance may be needed due to the location of the skin problem or the resident's physical or mental limitations.

Technique for Applying Topical Medications

Step 1: Wash your hands before and after application.

Step 2: Put on disposable gloves when applying an ointment, cream, lotion, solution, or shampoo directly to the skin. Use of gloves is especially important if you are applying medication to a wound or a reddened area of the skin.

Step 3: Do not apply directly with your fingers, and do not go back and forth between the medication container and the site of application—that may contaminate the medication container.

Step 4: Keep the area around the treatment site clean.

Step 5: Unless you are going to use the medication in the container only once, remove a small amount using a tongue depressor or something similar into a small disposable plastic or paper cup. Use that as your source for the medication to be applied to the skin. Discard whatever is left.

Step 6: When using cortisone-like products, a thin layer is adequate. Many of these topical preparations are very strong and require very little to achieve the therapeutic effect (many are also very expensive).

Step 7: Never lay opened, sterile bandages face down on anything but the wound, and always discard old dressings promptly outside the resident's room.

COMMON PROBLEMS

In every facility that provides assistance with medications, there will be situations that are out of the ordinary. Caregivers need to be able to anticipate these situations and respond appropriately.

Missed Doses

• When there is evidence that a resident who receives no assistance in administering medications frequently misses doses, it is a good indication that a reevaluation of the need for assistance is in order. Even when you are taking responsibility for reminding residents when to take medications or are actually preparing the doses, residents may still miss doses because they are unavailable at the time.

- Do not double up doses by administering twice as much at the next scheduled dose.

- Medications administered just once a day can usually be administered anytime that day. Do not double up the next day, however.

- If the dose is just an hour or two after the scheduled time, it should usually be administered at that time. If scheduled times are 4 hours or less apart and the dose is more than 2 hours late, it is usually better to skip that dose or the next dose, unless the drug is an antibiotic. If in doubt, check with the pharmacist.

- Directions for taking medications before and after meals are usually important to limit stomach or gastrointestinal discomfort or to increase absorption of the drug. If a missed dose is discovered too long after a meal, giving with a little food or milk will often be enough.

- Be sure to check with the resident's doctor or pharmacist if you are are unsure about what to do.

Wrong Dose or Wrong Medication

- Notify the resident's doctor immediately of any errors. Doses taken that are less than prescribed can easily be corrected by adding more medication to the dose taken. Excessive doses are not usually a serious problem, as long as the dose taken was not more than twice what was ordered. In most cases, there is simply a greater risk of side-effects such as dizziness or sedation. Wrong medications could have serious consequences. Except for allergies, a single dose of the wrong medication will not *usually* cause any significant or lasting harm, but contact the pharmacy or the resident's doctor in all cases.

Polypharmacy

- Polypharmacy is the word used to describe a resident who is taking many medications, often from several different doctors. When residents see several doctors, there can be problems if each doctor is not aware of what the others have prescribed. This can result in the use of drugs that interact with each other causing side-effects or in the use of two or more drugs that are very similar, resulting in an increased risk for side-effects. The solution is to be sure that each doctor is aware of the others' involvement (a difficult task if the resident is self-sufficient and visits the doctor and handles medications independently), and to be sure that the resident uses a pharmacy that maintains individual "patient profiles" so that the medicines prescribed by all the resident's doctors can be compared each time a new prescription is filled.

Cost

• Cost can be a major problem in drug therapy. Studies have shown that some prescriptions are not filled or refilled due to their cost. Although most facilities are not actually involved in purchasing medications, it may be helpful to talk with the doctor, who may be unaware of the problem and may be willing to prescribe a medication that is less expensive or is covered under a state Medicaid program or insurance plan. It may also be possible to negotiate better prices with the resident's pharmacy.

Compliance

• Some drug therapy may present compliance problems, either because the dosage form requires a certain amount of skill (for example, injectables like insulin, inhalers for breathing difficulties, or the insertion of vaginal suppositories), or because the results of the therapy are unpredictable. In these situations assistance should be provided only when not prohibited by state law and when the caregiver is certain of his or her skills. Doctors and pharmacists can offer advice and training information to increase skills, and information that will be helpful in monitoring the resident for side-effects.

• It is likely that, from time to time, you will have one or more residents who insist on using medications improperly, perhaps even to the point of abuse. This can range from addiction to narcotics or other drugs to overuse of nose drops. Whatever the reason, improper use of medications can result in resident discomfort, stress within the facility, and life-threatening side-effects. Although it is not your responsibility to cure this sort of behavior, it is important that the resident's doctors be aware of it. This is particularly true when a resident uses several different doctors—a common problem in individuals who overuse medications.

Side-Effects

- Caregivers are not expected to know all the side-effects of all the medications that residents take or even those with which they provide assistance. It is not unusual for the package insert of a prescription drug to list 50 to 60 potential side-effects. However, it is important to recognize when there is something different about a resident, and to have an awareness of at least the most likely or significant side-effects. The Medication Quick Reference lists the most commonly seen side-effects of the medications your residents are most likely to take. You should have at least one of the more comprehensive drug references listed in the appendix as well. Many pharmacies now include patient information leaflets when they dispense medications.

Many side-effects are mild and go away over time without making any changes. For example, if mild stomach or gastrointestinal discomfort is experienced (a common problem with drugs), it may be self-limiting or it may be resolved by giving the drug with food. Mental changes can also result from drug therapy. The pharmacy is a good source of information and guidance, as is the resident's doctor.

AUDITING YOUR CARE

Part of any successful system of care is the ability to define your residents' needs, to identify and resolve problems, and to use what you have learned to improve your care. This approach is part of current management concepts such as "total quality management." By now, you should be well on your way to creating a key portion of your review and improvement process—a well-defined set of policies and procedures that tell you and others how you intend to meet your residents' needs. Your audit and review process will focus first on how well those policies and procedures meet resident needs. You will then be able to determine if you need to reevaluate resident needs or the policies and procedures themselves, or if you simply need to make sure that the caregivers involved are properly trained and supervised.

The first step in an audit or review process is simply to evaluate your compliance with your own policies and procedures. This can be done with a yes–no checklist for each procedure, with explanatory comments added when you have checked "no" or at other appropriate times. If possible, use someone other than the person who routinely performs the functions you are checking. Some facilities may ask a pharmacist to assist. This inspection or review approach will tell you if the systems you have developed are in place and if caregivers are following procedures, at least at that time. What it cannot tell you is whether there are problems with your policies and procedures. Are your procedures too restrictive, and end up wasting time? Or are they inadequate in some area and do not afford your residents the level of service they need?

One way to determine how good your policies and procedures are is to keep track of problems that have been noted that relate to medications. For example, continued errors by staff may mean that medication assistance procedures are weak, not that the caregiver is inattentive or sloppy. Repeated resident visits to doctors or hospitals because of adverse drug reactions may indicate either errors in administration, a failure to monitor residents for potential problems, or the need for better policies and procedures if training and supervision are not the issue. In health facilities like hospitals or nursing facilities, these reports are referred to as "incident reports," and they are examined carefully to see what caused the problem.

Another way to measure your own performance is to list the resident outcomes you would like to see—such things as residents maintaining a positive mental attitude, eating well, sleeping well, maintaining their level of physical health, and so forth. When a comparison of your residents over time indicates failures that are not otherwise explained (such as a stroke, loss of loved one, etc.), look to see if there is a cause that may relate to the facility. Something as simple as a change in primary caregiver or the facility cook can make a big difference, as can improper administration of medications, or side-effects of medications. On the other hand, residents who are doing well offer a positive measure of your services.

After you have collected and analyzed information about your residents be prepared to make changes. Without that commitment, the rest of the process is just a waste of time.

THE MEDICATION QUICK REFERENCE (MQR)

There are over *eight thousand* different prescription and non-prescription drug names on the American market. Fortunately, RCF residents use only a small fraction of that number. The MQR lists that follow list only the medications you are most likely to see, and do not include very specialized or dangerous drugs such as those used for cancer treatment. However, doctors' prescribing habits vary greatly, and medications that are commonly prescribed in one community may never be seen in other areas. All drugs are listed in alphabetical order. When the generic name is listed in the first column, one or two brand names will be listed in the second column. If a brand name is listed first, the generic name will be listed in the second column. Generic drug names will always appear in italics. Brand names will always appear in red type. Detailed information about drug classifications appears in bold type.

How To Use the Medication Quick Reference

- Nearly all drugs have at least two names—the generic name and one or more brand names. In many cases we have listed the same medication in more than one location to make finding them easier.

- The effects and side-effects of similar drugs are cross-referenced so they can be found quickly. In some drug categories, each medication has about the same effects and side-effects as the others, and that information will be listed by drug class.

- This list of medications is not meant to be a complete reference. We have only listed what we think are the most common uses and the most important things you and your residents should watch for. Be sure to report side-effects to the doctor, and use more complete drug references when needed.

- For medications that are not listed, consult the resident's doctor or pharmacist or one of the more detailed references listed in the appendix.

- Most oral medications can cause stomach or gastrointestinal upset in anyone and skin rashes in people who are allergic to them, so these side-effects are not listed unless they are particularly significant.

- Side-effects often are more of a problem when therapy is first started or a dose is increased. In some cases, the body will adjust to these effects and they may no longer be seen after a few days or weeks.

- Always report any significant change in a resident to the resident's doctor, and be sure that the doctor is aware of *all* medications the resident is taking. For example, glaucoma medications, even though administered to the eye only, can sometimes have effects elsewhere in the body. These effects are called "systemic," and may include effects on blood pressure and pulse rate, among others. Also be sure the doctor who prescribes an antibiotic or other drug to treat an infection is aware of any medications or even foods to which the resident may be allergic.

- Refer to the section on routes and techniques for administration of medications for additional information on how to help residents with specific medications.

OTC Medications

The Medication Quick Reference list that follows includes the most common OTC drugs that your residents may be taking. Brand names are included only as examples, because listing all brand or trade names is not possible and all OTC drug labels include the medications' generic name(s).

It is important for you and the resident's doctor and pharmacist to be aware of all OTC medications a resident may be taking. It is also important for a resident not to take more than is recommended on the label unless ordered by the doctor.

Antacids: Antacids neutralize stomach acid. When stomach acid is excessive, it can cause stomach upset ("heartburn") and can contribute to the formation of stomach and duodenal ulcers. Antacids should be used carefully, because they can neutralize too much stomach acid and contribute to digestive problems; they can cause a "rebound" production of even more acid; and some cause constipation or diarrhea. Additionally, excessive use may indicate a problem other than stomach upset that should be addressed by a doctor. Other special concerns for antacids include the following.

- Antacids can cause changes in the body's absorption of other medications, so the resident's doctor or pharmacist should be aware of antacid use if the resident is also taking prescription medications.

- Some antacids, such as Tums, are commonly used to increase calcium intake, but they also retain their antacid effects regardless of their intended use.

- Most well-known antacids are a combination of more than one antacid. This helps to balance laxative and constipation effects. Many also include an anti-gas ingredient.

- Antacids only act locally (in the stomach and upper intestine). However, calcium, aluminum, and magnesium are absorbed into the bloodstream, and that absorption can result in both beneficial and harmful effects. It is especially important for residents with kidney disease to use these products only on a doctor's orders.

- As with most medicines, liquids work faster than tablets. If tablets are chewed well before swallowing, their effect is nearly as fast, and tablets are more convenient to carry. Be sure to let effervescent tablets dissolve completely before use.

Pain Medications (Analgesics): Pain medications are used for the relief of pain, fever, and sometimes inflammation or swelling. In some cases, the OTC drug is the same as the drug available by prescription only in a weaker strength. They can be harmful if used in excess of dosage directions on the label.

Cough and Cold Ingredients: It is important to check with the resident's doctor or pharmacist before using these products, especially if the resident has high blood pressure. Remember that coughing is a natural reflex to clear congestion from the lungs, so productive coughs (as opposed to dry, "hacking" coughs) should not be discouraged or prevented.

Eyedrops and Washes: Eye medications should always be used with caution. Always let the resident's doctor know if redness or discomfort continues. Do not use at the same time as prescription eye drops or ointments.

Laxatives: One of the most common health problems for elderly people is constipation. Usually, this problem can be resolved by eating a proper diet, including fruits and other foods with high fiber content, drinking plenty of fluids, and getting moderate exercise. Unfortunately, many older people use laxatives for "regularity," and develop what is often called a "laxative habit." In such cases, it may be possible to retrain bowel habits to lessen or eliminate the use of laxatives.

Constipation can lead to bowel obstruction, which can be very serious. When laxatives are required on a regular basis, however, it is best to use those with the least direct effect. Bulk laxatives such as Metamucil and stool softeners such as Colace come closest to mimicking the natural action of foods in promoting elimination. Bulk-producing laxatives can cause constipation, however, especially if given without adequate amounts of water or juice. Emollient or lubricant laxatives contain mineral oil in one form or another and work in a way similar to stool softeners. However, mineral oil can limit absorption of certain vitamins, and it is no longer widely used.

Medications that directly stimulate bowel movements by irritating the bowel are called irritant or stimulant laxatives. These medicines are not as desirable for long-term use, but are useful when a prompt effect is needed or when a person has lost the natural reflexes that promote elimination. Saline laxatives or cathartics act quickly and effectively by pulling water from the body into the intestines or, when used as an enema, from the colon. The effect is often similar to diarrhea and causes discomfort to the resident. Strong laxatives can cause a loss of important minerals that are either pulled into the intestine with body fluids or are not properly absorbed due to the speed with which the intestinal contents move through the colon. Some direct-action laxatives are used in combination with stool softeners.

Enemas act primarily by filling the colon, sometimes with just tap water, other times with liquids that draw in additional fluids, cause irritation, or are otherwise designed to cause rapid elimination. Enemas are usually reserved for situations in which other laxatives have failed.

Severe constipation often results from stool impactions, which must be removed by a health professional.

As with other OTC medications, do not hesitate to call the resident's doctor when laxatives are ineffective or when a resident is using medication more often than is usual or recommended.

Topical Antiseptics, Antibiotics, and Antifungal Agents: In OTC form, these products are intended for treatment of minor skin infections or as first aid to prevent infections. However, the OTC antibiotics and combinations of antibiotics are safe and very effective and are frequently prescribed by doctors. Allergies to these products are common, however, and rashes should be reported promptly to the resident's doctor and the medication discontinued until the doctor provides instructions.

Agents Used To Treat Scabies and Lice: It is important to follow directions exactly when using these medications. It is just as important to follow the recommended steps in washing clothing and bedding; otherwise the resident will become re-infected. These medications include lindane (Kwell), permethrin (Nix), and pyrethrins, which are included in many combination products.

MEDICATION QUICK REFERENCE

GENERIC AND BRAND NAME DRUGS		TREATMENT USES	CAREGIVER GUIDELINES
ASA	Aspirin (acetylsalicylic acid)	Relief of pain, inflammation, fever, prevention of strokes and heart attacks	Risk of GI irritation and ulcer. Can cause ringing in the ears. Shares side-effects with NSAIDs. See NSAID.
ACE inhibitors	**Accupril, Altace, Benazepril, Capoten, Captopril, Enalapril, Fosinopril, Lisinopril, Lotensin, Monopril, Prinivil, Quinapril, Ramipril, Vasotec, Zestril**	**Open up or dilate blood vessels, lowering blood pressure and easing the work of the heart High blood pressure, congestive heart failure, diabetic kidney disease**	**May cause swelling of the face or lips—if this occurs, call a doctor immediately. May also cause an annoying cough or tickle in the throat, an unpleasant taste in the mouth, loss of appetite, or light-headedness. Resident may require blood tests to make sure there are no problems.**
Accupril	*Quinapril*	High blood pressure, congestive heart failure	See ACE inhibitors.
Acetaminophen	Tylenol, *APAP*	Relief of pain, fever reduction	May cause severe or even fatal damage to the liver when taken in high doses. No more than 5 doses of two regular strength or 4 doses of extra strength should be taken per day. This means all medications with acetaminophen, including prescription and non-prescription medicines. Also available as suppository if resident is unable to take medication by mouth.
Acetaminophen with codeine (APAP with codeine)	Tylenol with codeine, Tylenol #2, #3, *APAP with codeine*	Relief of moderate to severe pain	May cause constipation, drowsiness, dizziness, confusion, nausea. Residents should avoid alcohol and use caution when taking other drugs that cause drowsiness.
Acetazolamide	Diamox	Glaucoma, edema, prevention of seizures	Give with food. May cause sun sensitivity, drowsiness. Report unusual pain, sore throat, fever, rash, bleeding, bruising, tingling, or tremors to doctor.
Acetophenazine	Tindal	Severe mental problems	See Antipsychotics.
Achromycin	*Tetracycline*	Antibiotic, infection	See Tetracycline.
Acular	*Ketorolac*	Relief of itching of the eye	See instructions for administering eye drops.

GENERIC AND BRAND NAME DRUGS		TREATMENT USES	CAREGIVER GUIDELINES
Adalat, Adalat CC	*Nifedipine*, Procardia	Angina, high blood pressure	See Calcium channel blockers. Adalat CC should be given on an empty stomach.
Adapin	*Doxepin*, Sinequan	Depression, anxiety	See Tricyclic antidepressants.
Adrenalin	*Epinephrine*	Asthma, allergy	See Epinephrine.
AeroBid	*Flunisolide*	Bronchial asthma, relieves broncho spasms	Usually given with other inhalers. Have resident use other inhalers at least 5 minutes before using AeroBid. Resident should rinse mouth with water after use. See instructions for inhaler use.
Afrin	*Oxymetazoline*	Stuffy nose	May cause rapid heart rate, loss of appetite, increased blood pressure.
Akineton	*Biperiden*	Parkinson's disease	See Anticholinergic drugs.
Albuterol	Proventil, Ventolin	Asthma, chronic obstructive pulmonary disease	See Bronchodilators.
Aldactazide	*Spironolactone Hydrochlorothiazide*	Hypertension, edema	See Aldactone and Hydrochlorothiazide.
Aldactone	*Spironolactone*	Hypertension, edema	May cause drowsiness, confusion, GI cramps, headache.
Aldomet	*Methyldopa*	High blood pressure	May cause low blood pressure and dizziness when standing up, sexual dysfunction, water retention, drowsiness, depression, headaches.
Alginic acid	Gaviscon	Heartburn, stomach ulcers	Usually given in combination with other antacids. Do not give with Tetracycline.
Allopurinol	Zyloprim	Gouty arthritis	May cause drowsiness, chills, fever, joint or muscle pain, sore throat, nausea or vomiting, skin rash. Do not take vitamin C without doctor's order.
Alprazolam	Xanax	Anxiety, agitation, panic disorder	See Benzodiazepines.
Altace	*Ramipril*	High blood pressure, congestive heart failure	See ACE inhibitors.

Italic = generic name   Red = brand name   Boldface = drug class information

Generic and Brand Name Drugs		Treatment Uses	Caregiver Guidelines
Aluminum carbonate gel	Basaljel	Heartburn, stomach ulcers	May cause constipation. See Antacids.
Aluminum hydroxide	Amphojel	Heartburn, stomach ulcers	May cause constipation. See Antacids.
Alupent	*Metaproterenol*	Chronic obstructive pulmonary disease (COPD), asthma	See Bronchodilators.
Amantadine	Symmetrel	Parkinson's disease, flu	May cause dizziness, headache, loss of appetite, nervousness, irritability, difficulty sleeping, blurred vision, urination problems, confusion, mental changes.
Ambenyl	*Bromodiphen-hydramine*	Allergies	May cause sedation, dry mouth, and blurred vision, especially in higher doses.
Ambien	*Zolpidem*	Insomnia	May cause headache, daytime drowsiness, memory loss. Residents should avoid alcohol and use caution when taking other drugs that cause drowsiness.
Amitriptyline	Elavil	Depression, sometimes pain	See Tricyclic antidepressants.
Amoxapine	Asendin	Depression	See Tricyclic antidepressants.
Amoxicillin	Amoxil	Antibiotic, infection	Related to penicillin. Note history or signs of allergic reactions such as rash or difficulty breathing. May cause stomach upset, diarrhea.
Amoxicillin-clavulanate	Augmentin	Antibiotic, infection	See Amoxicillin.
Ampicillin	Amcil, Polycillin	Antibiotic, infection	See Amoxicillin.
Anaprox	*Naproxen*	Relief of pain, inflammation	See NSAIDs.
Ancobon	*Flucytosine*	Fungus infection	May cause GI problems.
Anexsia	*Hydrocodone/APAP*	Relief of severe pain	See Narcotic analgesics.

GENERIC AND BRAND NAME DRUGS		TREATMENT USES	CAREGIVER GUIDELINES
Ansaid	*Flurbiprofen*	Pain, inflammation	See NSAID.
Anspor	*Cephradine*, Velosef	Antibiotic, infection	See Amoxicillin.
Anticholinergic Drugs	Akineton, Artane, Bentyl, *Benztropine, Biperiden*, Cogentin, *Cyproheptadine, Dicyclomine, Disopyramide,* Ditropan, Flavoxate, *Oxybutynin,* Periactin, Pro-Banthine, *Propantheline,* Urispas	**Blocks a type of nerve signal that goes to certain parts of the body.**	Use caution in heat (decreases sweating); may cause blurred vision, constipation, urinary retention, dry mouth, confusion, dizziness. Elderly persons are very sensitive to these effects. Use caution when antihistamines, antidepressants, antipsychotics are given together because of similar side-effects.
Antihistamines	Ambenyl, *Astemizole,* Benadryl, *Bromodiphenhydramine, Brompheniramine,* Chlor-Trimeton, *Chlorpheniramine, Clemastine, Cyproheptadine, Diphenhydramine,* Hismanal, Periactin, Phenergan, *Promethazine, Terfenadine*	Allergies. Most have anticholinergic effects that help in drying nasal secretions. Sedative side-effects (especially Benadryl) are used as night time sleep aids.	May cause sedation. Use caution when giving with other sedating drugs. See Anticholinergic drugs.
Antipsychotics	*Acetophenazine, Chlorpromazine, Clozapine*, Clozaril, Compazine, *Fluphenazine*, Haldol, *Haloperidol, Loxapine*, Loxitane, Mellaril, Moban, *Molindone*, Navane, *Perphenazine, Prochlorperazine,* Prolixin, *Promazine,* Risperdal, *Risperidone*, Sparine, *Thioridazine,* Thiothixene, Thorazine, Tindal, Trilifon	Control hallucinations, paronoia, delusions, and other disturbed thoughts in serious mental illnesses such as schizophrenia. They are also used in dementia patients, such as those with Alzheimer's disease.	May cause drowsiness, blurred vision, dry mouth, urinary retention, constipation, dizziness when standing up and possible falls, abnormal movement of lips, tongue, trunk, hands, and feet, shuffling gait, drooling, restless movements, slow blink rate of eyes, rigid body, tremors, difficulty moving, low blood pressure. May cause an increased sensitivity to the sun, sunburn occurs much more easily. Elderly persons are very sensitive to these effects.

Italic = generic name   Red = brand name   Boldface = drug class information

Generic and Brand Name Drugs		Treatment Uses	Caregiver Guidelines
Antivert	*Meclizine*	Motion sickness, vertigo	May cause drowsiness, restlessness, excitation, difficult urination, low blood pressure.
APAP	*Acetaminophen,* Tylenol	Relief of moderate to severe pain	See Acetaminophen.
Apresoline	*Hydralazine*	High blood pressure	May cause headaches, dizziness, diarrhea, irregular heartbeat, loss of appetite, chest pain, general discomfort or weakness, sore throat, fever, swelling, pain or numbness in joints, hands, or feet.
Artane	*Trihexyphenidyl*	Parkinson's disease	See Anticholinergic drugs.
Artificial tear sac	Lacrisert	Dry eyes	Long-acting artificial tear.
ASA/butalbital/ caffeine/codeine	Fiorinal with codeine	Relief of pain, especially headaches	See Narcotic analgesics.
Asendin	*Amoxapine*	Depression	See Tricyclic antidepressants.
Aspirin (acetylsalicylic acid)	ASA	Relief of pain, inflammation, to decrease risk of heart attack and stroke	Risk of GI irritation and ulcer in large doses. Available as suppository if resident unable to take pills. See NSAID.
Astemizole	Hismanal	Relief of allergy symptoms	May cause an increase in appetite. Be sure the doctor is aware of all other medications the resident is taking. Do not give this medication with grapefruit juice.
Atarax	*Hydroxyzine,* Vistaril	Itching, hay fever, allergies, anxiety, sedation	See Anticholinergic drugs and Antihistamines.
Atenolol	Tenormin	Angina, high blood pressure, irregular heartbeat, heart attack prevention	See Beta blockers.
Ativan	*Lorazepam*	Anxiety, insomnia	See Benzodiazepines.
Atropine	Found in eyedrops and Lomotil	Glaucoma, diarrhea, bowel cramps	See Anticholinergic drugs.
Attapulgite	Kaopectate	Stops or reduces diarrhea	Diarrhea can result in dehydration and loss of important minerals. Contact doctor if fever or diarrhea is severe or continues for more than a few days.

GENERIC AND BRAND NAME DRUGS		**TREATMENT USES**	**CAREGIVER GUIDELINES**
Atrovent	*Ipratropium*	Opens airways, increases air to lungs	See instructions for how to use an inhaler.
Augmentin	*Amoxicillin-clavulanate*	Antibiotic, infection	See Amoxicillin.
Aventyl	*Nortriptyline*	Depression	See Tricyclic antidepressants.
Axid	*Nizatidine*	Stomach and bowel ulcers, heartburn	See H-2 blockers.
Azithromycin	Zithromax	Antibiotic	Do not give with aluminum or magnesium antacids. See Clarithromycin.
Azmacort	*Triamcinolone*	Asthma	Have resident rinse mouth after use. See instructions for inhaler use.
Bacampicillin	Spectrobid	Antibiotic, infection	See Amoxicillin.
Baclofen	Lioresal	Muscle relaxant, facial pain	Give with food or milk. May cause dizziness, drowsiness. Do not stop taking drug abruptly.
Bactrim	Septra, *Trimethoprim/ sulphamethoxazole*	Antibiotic, infection	May cause rash. Encourage fluid intake.
Bactroban	*Mupirocin*	Skin infections	May cause rash, burning, itching.
Basaljel	*Aluminum carbonate gel, basic*	Antacid, ulcers, heartburn	May cause constipation.
Beclomethasone	Beclovent, Vanceril, Vancevase	Asthma	May cause nasal inflammation, chronic yeast infections. Residents should rinse mouth with water after using. See instructions for inhaler use.
Beepen VK	Betapen-VK, *Penicillin V, Penicillin VK*	Antibiotic, infection	See Amoxicillin.
Belladonna with Phenobarbital	Donnatal	Relief of bowel spasms	See Anticholinergics
Benadryl	Compoz, *Diphenhydramine,* Nytol, Sominex	Itching, anxiety, sedation, allergies	See Anticholinergic drugs and Antihistamines.
Benazepril	Lotensin	High blood pressure, congestive heart failure	See ACE inhibitors.

Italic = generic name   Red = brand name   Boldface = drug class information

GENERIC AND BRAND NAME DRUGS		TREATMENT USES	CAREGIVER GUIDELINES
Benemid	*Probenecid*	Gouty arthritis	May cause headache, loss of appetite, blood in urine, painful urination, lower back or side pain. Residents should avoid alcohol and aspirin during treatment. Encourage lots of water, especially at first.
Bentyl	*Dicyclomine*	Relief of bowel spasms	See Anticholinergic drugs.
Benzocaine	Americaine	Local anesthetic, reduces pain and itching	May cause numbness.
Benzodiazepines	*Alprazolam,* Ativan, Centrax, *Chlordiazepoxide, Clonazepam, Clorazepate,* Dalmane, *Diazepam, Estazolam, Flurazepam,* Halazepam, Halcion, Klonopin, Librium, *Lorazepam,* Paxipam, *Prazepam,* ProSom, *Temazepam,* Tranxene, *Triazolam,* Valium	**Anxiety, agitation, insomnia, sometimes used for relief of muscle spasms and seizure control**	**May cause loss of memory, poor balance, dizziness, loss of concentration, confusion, depression, irritability, trouble sleeping. May be habit forming. Residents should avoid alcohol and use caution when taking other drugs that cause drowsiness. Can cause irritability, nervousness, and insomnia when dosage is lowered. The elderly are very sensitive to the effects of these drugs. Every night use for insomnia should be avoided.**
Benztropine	Cogentin	Parkinson's disease	See Anticholinergic drugs.
Bepridil	Vascor	Angina	See Calcium channel blockers.
Beta blockers	*Atenolol, Carteolol,* Cartrol, Corgard, Inderal, *Labetalol,* Lopressor, *Metoprolol, Nadolol,* Normodyne, *Pindolol, Propranolol,* Tenormin, *Timolol,* Trandate, Visken	**Help to lower heart rate and ease the work of the heart muscle, thereby helping to lower blood pressure and control or prevent heart rhythm abnormalities. Angina, high blood pressure, irregular heartbeat, prevention of heart attack.**	**May cause a too-dramatic lowering of blood pressure or a too-slow heart rate as well as breathing difficulties (especially in asthma). May also cause low blood sugar, confusion, hallucinations, cold hands or feet, depression, nightmares, or swelling in lower extremities. Residents should avoid alcohol and use caution when taking other drugs that cause drowsiness.**
Betagan	*Levobunolol*	Glaucoma	See instructions for administering eye drops.

Generic and Brand Name Drugs		Treatment Uses	Caregiver Guidelines
Bethanechol	Urecholine	Excessive urinary retention in bladder	May cause nausea, vomiting, diarrhea, abdominal cramps, flushing. Give 1 hour before or 2 hours after meals.
Biaxin	*Clarithromycin*	Antibiotic, infection	See Clarithromycin.
Biperiden	Akineton	Parkinson's disease	See Anticholinergic drugs.
Bisacodyl	Dulcolax	Stimulant laxative	Do not crush tablets or give with antacids or milk.
Bismuth subsalicylate	Pepto-Bismol	Diarrhea	Also used for indigestion, nausea, some abdominal cramps.
Bleph-10	*Sodium sulfacetamide,* Sulamyd	Eye infections	May sensitize eye to bright light. See instructions for administering eye drops.
Blocadren	*Timolol*	Prevention of hypertension, heart attack, migraine	See Beta blockers.
Bromocriptine	Parlodel	Parkinson's disease	May cause nausea and drowsiness at beginning of therapy, low blood pressure, dizziness, nightmares, insomnia, hallucinations. Residents should avoid alcohol and use caution when taking other drugs that cause drowsiness. Give with food or milk.
Bromodiphenhydramine	Ambenyl	Allergies	See Antihistamines.
Brompheniramine	Dimetane	Allergies, cold symptoms	See Antihistamines.
Bronchodilators	*Albuterol,* **Alupent,** *Metaproterenol,* **Proventil, Ventolin**	**Help to relax the airways and ease the work of breathing, thereby promoting improved ventilation of the lungs. Chronic obstructive pulmonary disease, asthma**	**May cause rapid heart rate, tremor, nervousness, or insomnia.**

Italic = generic name   Red = brand name   Boldface = drug class information

GENERIC AND BRAND NAME DRUGS		TREATMENT USES	CAREGIVER GUIDELINES
Bumex	*Bumetanide*	High blood pressure, congestive heart failure, edema	See Diuretics.
Bupropion	Wellbutrin	Depression	May cause weight loss, dizziness, agitation, anxiety, seizures, confusion, tremors, insomnia, restlessness. Residents should avoid alcohol.
BuSpar	*Buspirone*	Anxiety, depression, behavior problems in dementia patients	May cause lightheadedness, dizziness, headache, excitement, restlessness. Residents should avoid alcohol and use caution when taking other drugs that cause drowsiness.
Calan	Isoptin, *Verapamil*	High blood pressure, angina, irregular heartbeat	See Calcium channel blockers.
Calcium carbonate	Tums	Antacid	Give with food if used to increase calcium intake.
Calcium channel blockers	**Adalat, Adalat CC, Bepridil, Calan, Calan SR, Cardene, Cardizem, Cardizem SR, Dilacor, Dilacor XR, *Diltiazem*, DynaCirc, *Felodipine*, Isoptin, Isoptin SR, Isradipine, *Nicardipine*, *Nifedipine*, Plendil, Procardia, Vascor, *Verapamil***	**Dilate the coronary arteries and reduce the work of the heart. Help prevent or control abnormal heart rhythms. Angina, high blood pressure, irregular heartbeat Raynaud's disease**	**May cause gum tenderness and bleeding, fast or slow heart rate, swelling in the lower extremities, dizziness, headache, flushing or a warm feeling.**
Capoten	*Captopril*	High blood pressure, congestive heart failure	See ACE inhibitor.
Capsaicin	Zostrix	Relieves pain from arthritis, shingles, other local nerve pain	Avoid contact with eyes and mouth. Wash hands immediately after applying. May cause a burning feeling at application site.

GENERIC AND BRAND NAME DRUGS		TREATMENT USES	CAREGIVER GUIDELINES
Carafate	*Sucralfate*	Stomach and bowel ulcers	May cause constipation, drowsiness. Give with water 1 hour before meals. Give no antacids for 30 minutes. Do not give with the following drugs: Enoxacin, Lomefloxin, Norfloxacin, or Ofloxacin.
Carbachol	Isopto Carbachol	Glaucoma	See instructions for administering eye drops.
Carbamazepine	Tegretol	Seizures, facial pain	May cause increased sensitivity to sun, vision or eye movement problems, unusual bleeding or bruising, light-colored stools, drowsiness, dizziness, mouth sores.
Carbenicillin	Geocillin, Geopen	Antibiotic, infection	See Amoxicillin.
Cardene	*Nicardipine*	Angina, high blood pressure, congestive heart failure	See Calcium channel blockers.
Cardizem, Cardizem SR	Dilacor, Dilacor XR, *Diltiazem*	Angina, Raynaud's disease	See Calcium channel blockers.
Carteolol	Cartrol, Ocupress	Glaucoma, high blood pressure, angina	See Beta blockers and instructions for administering eye drops.
Casanthranol	Peri-Colace	Constipation	Stimulant laxative.
Catapres	*Clonidine*	High blood pressure	Comes as pills or a patch. Do not put patch on reddened area or broken skin; date patch, rotate site, and check placement daily. Be sure to use medicated patch, not just protective cover. May cause drowsiness, dizziness when standing up, dry mouth, depression, edema. Do not discontinue abruptly. See instructions for applying patch.
Ceclor	*Cefaclor*	Antibiotic, infection	See Amoxicillin.
Cefadroxil	Duricef, Ultracef	Antibiotic, infection	See Amoxicillin.

Italic = generic name Red = brand name Boldface = drug class information

GENERIC AND BRAND NAME DRUGS		TREATMENT USES	CAREGIVER GUIDELINES
Cefixime	Suprax	Antibiotic, infection	See Amoxicillin.
Cefpodoxime	Vantin	Antibiotic, infection	See Amoxicillin.
Cefprozil	Cefzil	Antibiotic, infection	See Amoxicillin.
Ceftin	*Cefuroxime*	Antibiotic, infection	See Amoxicillin.
Cephalexin	Cefanex, Keflex	Antibiotic, infection	See Amoxicillin.
Cephradine	Anspor, Velosef	Antibiotic, infection	See Amoxicillin.
Cephulac	Chronulac, *Lactulose*	Liver disease, chronic constipation	May cause gas, belching. Do not give with antacids.
Chlor-Trimeton	*Chlorpheniramine*	Itching, hayfever, allergies	May cause drowsiness, dizziness, confusion, hallucinations. Residents should avoid alcohol and use caution when taking other drugs that cause drowsiness. See Anticholinergic drugs.
Chloral hydrate	Noctec	Insomnia	May cause excess drowsiness, confusion, headache, nausea, gas. May be habit forming. Residents should avoid alcohol and use caution when taking other drugs that cause drowsiness.
Chloramphenicol	Chloroptic	Antibiotic, eye infections	See instructions for administering eye drops.
Chlordiazepoxide	Librium	Anxiety	Caution should be taken when giving medication to elderly residents due to long-lasting effects and the increased risk of falls. See Benzodiazepines.
Chloroptic	*Chloramphenicol*	Antibiotic, eye infections	See instructions for administering eye drops.
Chlorpheniramine	Chlor-Trimeton	Itching, hay fever, allergies	See Antihistamines.
Chlorpromazine	Thorazine	Severe mental problems	See Antipsychotics.
Chlorthalidone	Hygroton	High blood pressure, congestive heart failure, edema	See Diuretics.

GENERIC AND BRAND NAME DRUGS		TREATMENT USES	CAREGIVER GUIDELINES
Chlorzoxazone	Parafon Forte	Muscle relaxant	May cause dizziness, urine may turn orange or purple. Residents should avoid alcohol and use caution when taking other drugs that cause drowsiness. Give with food or milk.
Choledyl	*Oxytriphylline*	Increases air flow to lungs	See Theophylline.
Cholestyramine	Cholybar, Questran	Lowers blood cholesterol	May cause severe constipation, sudden weight loss.
Choline magnesium salicylate	Trilisate	Pain, inflammation	See NSAID.
Chronulac	Cephulac, *Lactulose*	Liver disease, chronic constipation	May cause gas, belching. Do not give with antacids.
Ciloxan	*Ciprofloxacin*	Eye infection	See instructions for administering eye drops.
Cimetidine	Tagamet	Stomach and bowel ulcers, heartburn	See H-2 blockers.
Cipro	*Ciprofloxacin*	Antibiotic, infection	See Ciprofloxacin.
Ciprofloxacin	Cipro	Antibiotic, infection	Use caution in residents with seizure disorders or who take Theophylline. Do not give antacids, zinc, iron, or the drug Carafate with this drug or 4 hours before or 2 hours after taking this drug. Minimize exposure to the sun.
Clarithromycin	Biaxin	Antibiotic, infection	May cause diarrhea, nausea, stomach upset, and headache. It can cause reactions with many drugs. Make sure the doctor knows all medications the resident is taking.
Clemastine	Tavist D	Hay fever, allergies, itching	See Antihistimines.
Cleocin	*Clindamycin,* Dalacin C	Antibiotic, infection	Contact doctor if resident develops diarrhea.
Clindamycin	Cleocin, Dalacin C	Antibiotic, infection	Contact doctor if resident develops diarrhea.

Italic = generic name   Red = brand name   Boldface = drug class information

GENERIC AND BRAND NAME DRUGS		TREATMENT USES	CAREGIVER GUIDELINES
Clonazepam	Klonopin	Seizures (epilepsy), behavior control	Use caution when giving medication to elderly residents due to long-lasting effects and the possibility of falls. See Benzodiazepines.
Clonidine	Catapres	High blood pressure	See Catapres.
Clorazepate	Tranxene	Anxiety	See Benzodiazepines.
Clotrimazole	Gyne-Lotrimin	Vaginal infections	Use vaginal applicator if so directed.
Cloxacillin	Tegopen	Antibiotic, infection	See Amoxicillin.
Clozapine	Clozaril	Severe mental disorders	See Antipsychotics. Resident will need to have weekly blood testing.
Cogentin	*Benztropine*	Parkinson's disease and other movement disorders	See Anticholinergic drugs.
Cognex	*Tacrine*	Improves mental capabilities, slows progression of mild to moderate dementia of Alzheimer's disease	May cause nausea, vomiting, diarrhea. Give before meals. OK to take with meals if resident develops upset stomach. Resident will need regular lab tests.
Colace	*Docusate sodium, DSS, DOS*	Constipation, stool softener	Useful only if adequate fluid in diet. High in salt content; can cause swelling of the ankles.
Colestid	*Colestipol*	Lowers blood cholesterol	May cause severe constipation, weight loss.
Compazine	*Prochlorperazine*	Vomiting, nausea	See Antipsychotics.
Conjugated estrogen	Premarin	Estrogen for replacement therapy, prevention of osteoporosis	May cause sudden severe headache, vomiting, visual or speech disturbances, shortness of breath, chest pain, depression, unusual bleeding.
Corgard	*Nadolol*	High blood pressure	See Beta blockers.
Coumadin	*Warfarin*	Anticoagulant (blood thinner)	Call doctor immediately if resident develops unusual bleeding or bruising. Notify other doctors of all other medicines resident is taking.
Cyclobenzaprine	Flexeril	Muscle relaxant	See Flexeril.

GENERIC AND BRAND NAME DRUGS		TREATMENT USES	CAREGIVER GUIDELINES
Cyproheptadine	Periactin	Allergies, appetite stimulation	See Antihistamines.
Cytotec	*Misoprostol*	Prevents stomach ulcers caused by NSAIDs	May cause headache, abdominal pain, gas, and diarrhea.
Cytovene	*Ganciclovir*	Viral eye infection	See instructions for administering eye drops.
Dalmane	*Flurazepam*	Insomnia	Use caution when giving medication to elderly residents due to long-lasting effects and the possibility of falls. See **Benzodiazepines**.
Dantrolene	Dantrium	Muscle relaxant	May cause sun sensitivity, drowsiness, dizziness, headache, muscle weakness.
Daypro	*Oxaprozin*	Pain, arthritis	See **NSAID**.
Darvocet-N	*Propoxyphene N with APAP*	Pain relief	May cause drowsiness, dizziness, blurred vision, excitement, insomnia. See **Narcotic analgesics**.
Decadron	*Dexamethasone*	Reduces inflammation	See Prednisone.
Declomycin	*Demeclocycline*	Antibiotic, infection	Related to Tetracycline. Watch for sun sensitivity reaction. See **Tetracycline**.
Demecarium	Humorsol	Glaucoma	See instructions for administering eye drops.
Demeclocycline	Declomycin	Antibiotic, also used for disorders of salt content of the blood	Related to Tetracycline. Watch for sun sensitivity reaction. See **Tetracycline**.
Demerol	*Meperidine*	Relief of severe pain	See **Narcotic analgesics**.
Depakene	*Valproic acid*	Seizures (epilepsy); behavior modification in selected cases	May cause drowsiness, tremor, unsteadiness, confusion, restlessness, dizziness, sore throat, fever, fatigue. Give with food or milk. If resident has trouble swallowing capsule, open and mix contents with soft food that can be swallowed without chewing.

Italic = generic name   Red = brand name   Boldface = drug class information

GENERIC AND BRAND NAME DRUGS		TREATMENT USES	CAREGIVER GUIDELINES
Depakote	Depakene, *Divalproex*, Valproic acid	See Depakane	See Depakane
Desipramine	Norpramin	Depression	See Tricyclic antidepressants.
Desyrel	*Trazodone*	Depression, insomnia; behavior problems in dementia patients	May cause light-headedness especially when first standing up, confusion, falls. See Tricylic antidepressants
Dexamethasone	Decadron	Reduces inflammation	See Prednisone.
Dextromethorphan	Robitussin-DM	Cough suppressant	May cause confusion or constipation in high doses.
DiaBeta	*Glyburide*, Micronase	Diabetes	Can cause low blood sugar. See Glipizide.
Diazepam	Valium	Anxiety, muscle relaxant, seizures	Use caution when giving medication to elderly residents due to long-lasting effects and the possibility of falls. See Benzodiazepines.
Diclofenac	Voltaren	Pain, inflammation	See NSAID.
Dicloxacillin	Dynapen	Antibiotic, infection	See Amoxicillin.
Dicyclomine	Bentyl	GI spasm	See Anticholinergic drugs.
Digoxin	Lanoxin	Congestive heart failure, irregular heartbeat	May cause low pulse rate, lack of appetite, nausea.
Dilacor, Dilacor XR	Cardizem, Cardizem SR, *Diltiazem*	Angina, Raynaud's disease	XR is an extended release form See Calcium channel blockers.
Dilantin	*Phenytoin*	Seizures (epilepsy)	May cause drowsiness, vision problems, unsteadiness.
Dilaudid	*Hydromorphone*	Relief of severe pain	See Narcotic analgesics.
Diltiazem	Cardizem, Cardizem SR, Dilacor, Dilacor XR	Angina, Raynaud's disease	See Calcium channel blockers.
Diphenhydramine	Benadryl	Itching, allergies, sedation	See Antihistimines.

GENERIC AND BRAND NAME DRUGS		TREATMENT USES	CAREGIVER GUIDELINES
Diphenoxylate/ atropine	Lomotil	Diarrhea	May cause drowsiness, dizziness, dry mouth, constipation. Residents should avoid alcohol and use caution when taking other drugs that cause drowsiness.
Dipyridamole	Persantine	Prevents blood clots, increases blood flow to the heart	May cause dizziness, flushing, increased bruising or bleeding.
Disalcid	*Salsalate*	Pain, inflammation	See NSAID.
Disopyramide	Norpace	Irregular heartbeat	May cause chest pains, irregular heartbeat, nervousness, dizziness. See Anticholinergic drugs.
Ditropan	*Oxybutynin*	Urinary spasms	See Anticholinergic drugs.
Diuretics	***Bumetanide*, Bumex, *Chlorthalidone*, Dyazide, *Furosemide*, *Hydrochlorothi-azide*, Hydrodiuril, Hygroton, *Indapamide*, Lasix, Lozol, Maxzide**	**Increases the elimination of water and salt in the urine. High blood pressure, congestive heart failure, edema**	**May cause loss of potassium and dizziness when standing up, increased sensitivity to sunburn. Do not give in the evening unless ordered by the doctor. Residents should avoid alcohol and use caution when taking other drugs that cause drowsiness.**
Divalproex	Depakote, Depakane, Valproic acid	Seizures	See Depakote.
Docusate calcium and sodium	Surfak (calcium) Colace, DSS, DOS (sodium)	Constipation	Stool softener. Useful only if adequate fluid in diet.
Donnatal	*Belladonna*	Relief of bowel spasms	See Anticholinergics
Doxepin	Adapin, Sinequan	Depression, anxiety	See Tricyclic antidepressants.
Doxycycline	Doryx, Vibramycin	Antibiotic, infection	See Tetracycline.
Duragesic (patch)	*Fentanyl*	Severe, chronic pain	Use with caution and dispose of safely. Rotate sites. See Narcotic analgesics. See instructions for applying patch.

Italic = generic name   Red = brand name   Boldface = drug class information

GENERIC AND BRAND NAME DRUGS		TREATMENT USES	CAREGIVER GUIDELINES
Duricef	*Cefadroxil,* Ultracef	Antibiotic, infection	See Amoxicillin.
Dyazide	Maxzide, *Triamterene/ hydrochlorothiazide*	High blood pressure, edema (swelling)	See Diuretics.
DynaCirc	*Isradipine*	High blood pressure	See Calcium channel blockers.
Dynapen	*Dicloxacillin*	Antibiotic, infections	See Amoxicillin.
Echothiophate	Phospholine Iodide	Glaucoma	See Phospholine Iodide.
Effexor	*Venlafaxine*	Depression	May cause insomnia, nervousness, anxiety, tremor, sweating, loss of appetite, sexual dysfunction, drowsiness, weakness.
Elavil	*Amitriptyline*	Depression, sometimes pain	See Tricyclic antidepressants.
Eldepryl	*Selegiline*	Parkinson's disease	May cause dizziness, severe headache, hallucinations, depression, insomnia, involuntary movements, irregular heartbeat.
Elixophyllin	*Theophylline*	Increases air to lungs	See Theophylline.
Enalapril	Vasotec	High blood pressure, congestive heart failure	See ACE inhibitors.
Encainide	Enkaid	Irregular heartbeat	May cause chest pain, irregular heartbeat, dizziness, headache, insomnia, nervousness, cough.
Enkaid	*Encainide*	Irregular heartbeat	See Encainide.
Enoxacin	Penetrex	Antibiotic, infection	Do not administer with Carafate (sucralfate), antacids, zinc, or iron. See Ciprofloxacin.
Ephedrine	Efedron	Runny nose, nasal congestion	May cause headache, nervousness, insomnia, rapid heart rate, elevated blood pressure.
Epinephrine (inhaler)	Adrenalin	Asthma, allergy	May cause headache, nervousness, rapid heart rate.

GENERIC AND BRAND NAME DRUGS		TREATMENT USES	CAREGIVER GUIDELINES
Erythromycin	Erythrocin, Ilotycin	Antibiotic, infection	May cause upset stomach. See Clarithromycin.
Eserine	*Physostigmine*	Glaucoma	See instructions for administering eye drops.
Estazolam	ProSom	Insomnia	See Benzodiazepines.
Estradiol	Estrace, Estraderm patch	Estrogen replacement therapy, prevention of osteoporosis	May cause sudden severe headache, vomiting, visual or speech disturbance, shortness of breath, chest pain, depression, unusual bleeding.
Etodolac	Lodine	Pain, inflammation	See NSAID.
Euthroid	*Liotrix*	Thyroid hormone	May cause chest pain, weight loss, nervousness, fast heartbeat, sweating, and insomnia.
Famvir	*Famciclovir*	Shingles	May cause headache, upset stomach.
Famotidine	Pepcid	Stomach and bowel ulcers, heartburn	See H-2 blockers.
Feldene	*Piroxicam*	Inflammation, pain	See NSAID.
Felodipine	Plendil	High blood pressure	See Calcium channel blockers.
Fentanyl	Duragesic patch	Severe, chronic pain	See Duragesic and Narcotic analgesics.
Finasteride	Proscar	Prostrate enlargement	If tablets are crushed the powder can cause birth defects if touched or inhaled by a pregnant woman.
Fiorinal with codeine	*ASA/butalbital caffeine/codeine*	Pain relief	See Narcotic analgesics.
Flavoxate	Urispas	Urinary bladder spasms that cause incontinence	See Anticholinergic drugs.
Flecainide	Tambocor	Irregular heartbeat	May cause irregular heartbeat, dizziness, fatigue, tremor, nervousness, headache.

Italic = generic name   Red = brand name   Boldface = drug class information

Generic and Brand Name Drugs		Treatment Uses	Caregiver Guidelines
Flexeril	*Cyclobenzaprine*	Muscle relaxant	May cause drowsiness, dizziness, blurred vision. Residents should avoid alcohol and other sedating drugs.
Floxin	*Ofloxacin*	Antibiotic	See Ciprofloxacin.
Fluorometholone	FML	Reduces eye inflammation	See instructions for administering eye drops.
Fluoxetine	Prozac	Depression, obsessive–compulsive disorder	See Prozac.
Fluphenazine	Prolixin	Severe mental problems	See Antipsychotics.
Flurazepam	Dalmane	Insomnia	Use caution when giving medication to elderly residents due to long-lasting effects and the possibility of falls. See Benzodiazepines.
Flurbiprofen	Ansaid	Pain, inflammation	See NSAID.
Flurbiprofen sodium	Ocufen	Reduces eye inflammation	May cause stinging and burning of the eyes. See instructions for administering eye drops.
Fluvastatin	Lescol	Lowers blood cholesterol	May cause GI problems, headache. Give with meals.
FML	*Fluorometholone*	Reduces eye inflammation	See instructions for administering eye drops.
Foscavir	*Foscarnet*	Viral infections of eye	See instructions for administering eye drops.
Fosinopril	Monopril	High blood pressure	See ACE inhibitors.
Furosemide	Lasix	High blood pressure, fluid edema, congestive heart failure	Water pill causes increased urination, may precipitate urinary incontinence, may cause dizziness, may trigger gout. See Diuretics.
Ganciclovir	Cytovene	Viral infection of eye	See instructions for administering eye drops.
Gantrisin	*Sulfisoxazole*	Antibiotic, infection	Can cause rash, fever, confusion.

GENERIC AND BRAND NAME DRUGS		TREATMENT USES	CAREGIVER GUIDELINES
Garamycin	*Gentamycin*	Antibiotic, infections of the eye	See instructions for administering eye drops.
Gemfibrozil	Lopid	Lowers blood cholesterol	See Lopid.
Gentamycin	Garamycin	Antibiotic, infections of the eye	See instructions for administering eye drops.
Geocillin, Geopen	*Carbenicillin*	Antibiotic, infection	See Amoxicillin.
Glipizide	Glucotrol	Diabetes	May cause dangerously low blood sugar, especially if meals are skipped. If resident is skipping meals while on this drug, call doctor. If confusion or change in personality, offer juice or candy and call doctor.
Glucophage	*Metformin*	Diabetes	Notify doctor immediately if excessive sleepiness, trouble breathing, or general illness develops or if resident's food or fluid intake decreases significantly.
Glucotrol	Glipizide	Diabetes	See Glipizide.
Glyburide	DiaBeta, Micronase	Diabetes	See Glipizide.
Guanfacine	Tenex	High blood pressure	May cause dizziness, drowsiness, headache. Give at bedtime.
Guiafenesin	Robitussin	Cough, expectorant which loosens respiratory secretions.	May cause nausea.
H-2 blockers	**Axid, Cimetidine, Famotidine, Nizatidine, Pepcid, Ranitidine, Tagamet, Zantac**	**Stomach and bowel ulcers, heartburn. Decrease acidity in the stomach by blocking normal acid-production mechanisms.**	**May cause diarrhea, dizziness, drowsiness, headache, and muscle aches. These medications should be taken with or just after meals and not with antacids. Be sure doctor is aware of all medications that resident is taking.**
Halazepam	Paxipam	Anxiety	See Benzodiazepines.
Halcion	*Triazolam*	Insomnia	May cause loss of memory of recent events. See Benzodiazepines.

Italic = generic name Red = brand name Boldface = drug class information

GENERIC AND BRAND NAME DRUGS		TREATMENT USES	CAREGIVER GUIDELINES
Haldol	*Haloperidol*	Severe mental problems	See Antipsychotics.
Haloperidol	Haldol	Severe mental problems	See Antipsychotics.
Herplex	*Idoxuridine*	Herpes infection of the eye	See instructions for administering eye drops.
Hismanal	*Astemizole*	Relief of allergy symptoms	May cause an increase in appetite. It has many drug interactions—be sure the doctor is aware of all other medications the resident is taking. Do not take this drug with grapefruit juice.
HMS	*Medrysone*	Reduces inflammation	See instructions for administering eye drops.
Homatropine	Many brands	Glaucoma	See instructions for administering eye drops.
Humorsol	*Demecarium*	Glaucoma	See instructions for administering eye drops.
Hydralazine	Apresoline	High blood pressure	May cause headaches, dizziness, diarrhea, irregular heartbeat, loss of appetite, chest pain, general discomfort or weakness, sore throat, fever, swelling, pain or numbness in joints, hands, or feet.
Hydrochlorothiazide (HCTZ)	Hydrodiuril	High blood pressure, edema, congestive heart failure	See Diuretics.
Hydrocodone and Acetaminophen	Lortab , Vicodin	Relief of pain	See Narcotic analgesics.
Hydrocortisone	Many brands of ointments and creams	Reduces inflammation, swelling, itching	May increase severity of some infections. Can be absorbed from open wound or abrasion.
Hydrodiuril	*Hydrochlorothiazide*	See Hydrochlorothiazide	See Diuretics.
Hydromorphone	Dilaudid	Relief of severe pain	See Narcotic analgesics.
Hydroxyzine	Atarax, Vistaril	Itching, anxiety, sedation	May cause drowsiness, dizziness, confusion, hallucinations. Residents should avoid alcohol and use caution when taking other drugs that cause drowsiness. See Anticholinergic drugs.

GENERIC AND BRAND NAME DRUGS		TREATMENT USES	CAREGIVER GUIDELINES
Hygroton	*Chlorthalidone*	High blood pressure, congestive heart failure, edema	See Diuretics.
Hyoscine	Many brands	Glaucoma	See instructions for administering eye drops.
Hytrin	*Terazosin*	High blood pressure, prostate enlargement	May cause low blood pressure, dizziness and fainting when getting up, especially with first dose.
Ibuprofen	Motrin, Motrin IB, Advil	Pain, inflammation, arthritis, fever	See NSAID.
Idoxuridine	Herplex	Herpes infections of the eye	See instructions for administering eye drops.
Imipramine	Tofranil	Depression	See Tricyclic antidepressants.
Imodium	Imodium AD, *Loperimide*	Diarrhea	May cause drowsiness, dry mouth, dizziness, constipation. If diarrhea continues for 2 to 3 days, call doctor.
Indapamide	Lozol	High blood pressure, edema, heart failure	See Diuretics.
Inderal	*Propranolol*	High blood pressure, angina, irregular heartbeat, tremors	See Beta blockers.
Indocin	*Indomethacin*	Inflammation, pain	See NSAID.
Ipratropium	Atrovent	Opens airways, increases air to lungs	See instructions for how to use an inhaler.
Isoptin, Isoptin SR	Calan, Calan SR, *Verapamil*	High blood pressure, angina, irregular heartbeat	See Calcium channel blockers.
Isosorbide dinitrate	Isordil, Sorbitrate	Angina, congestive heart failure, esophagus spasm	May cause low blood pressure and possible falls when standing up after sitting; headache, rapid heartbeat, flushing.
Isradipine	DynaCirc	High blood pressure	See Calcium channel blockers.

Italic = generic name   Red = brand name   Boldface = drug class information

GENERIC AND BRAND NAME DRUGS		TREATMENT USES	CAREGIVER GUIDELINES
K-Dur, K-Tab, Kaon, KCL	*Potassium chloride,* Micro K, Slow-K	Potassium supplement	May cause nausea, vomiting, diarrhea, gas, abdominal discomfort. KCL liquid has a bitter taste.
Keflex	Cefanex, *Cephalexin,* Keftab	Antibiotic, infections	Allergic reactions may occur in residents with penicillin allergy. See Amoxicillin.
Ketoprofen	Orudis	Pain, inflammation	See NSAID.
Ketorolac	Acular, Toradol	Relief of allergic itching of the eye, pain	See instructions for administering eye drops. See NSAID.
Klonopin	*Clonazepam*	Seizures (epilepsy), agitation, anxiety, movement disorders	Use caution when giving medication to elderly residents due to long-lasting effects and the possibility of falls. See Benzodiazepines.
Labetalol	Normodyne, Trandate	High blood pressure	See Beta blockers.
Lacrisert	*Artificial tear sac*	Eye lubricant	Long-acting artificial tear application.
Lactulose	Cephulac, Chronulac	Liver disease, chronic constipation	May cause gas, belching. Do not give with antacids.
Lanoxin	*Digoxin*	Congestive heart failure, irregular heartbeat	May cause low pulse rate, lack of appetite, nausea.
Lasix	*Furosemide*	High blood pressure, fluid, edema, congestive heart failure	See Furosemide. See Diuretics.
Lescol	*Fluvastatin*	Lowers blood cholesterol	May cause GI problems, headache. Give with meals.
Levatol	*Penbutolol*	Irregular heartbeat	See Beta blockers.
Levobunolol	Betagan	Glaucoma	See instructions for administering eye drops.
Levocabastine	Livostin	Reduces allergic inflammation of the eye	See instructions for administering eye drops.
Levodopa/carbidopa	Sinemet	Parkinson's disease	May cause anxiety, insomnia, nervousness, hallucinations, fast or fluttering heartbeat, low blood pressure when standing up; increase risk of falls. Give on empty stomach unless stomach problems.

Generic and Brand Name Drugs		Treatment Uses	Caregiver Guidelines
Levothyroxine	Levothroid, Synthroid	Thyroid replacement therapy	May cause chest pain, weight loss, nervousness, rapid heartbeat, sweating, insomnia.
Librium	*Chlordiazepoxide*	Anxiety, agitation	See Chlordiazepoxide.
Lincomycin	Lincocin	Antibiotic, infection	May cause GI distress given 1 hour before or 2 hours after meal.
Lioresal	*Baclofen*	Muscle relaxant, spasms, facial pain	See Baclofen.
Lisinopril	Prinivil, Zestril	High blood pressure, congestive heart failure	See ACE inhibitors.
Lithium	Lithane	Manic–depression	May cause tremors, confusion, drowsiness, weakness, headache, irregular heart rate. Dangerous if blood levels too high. Alert doctor if resident is taking diuretics.
Livostin	*Levocabastine*	Reduces allergic inflammation of the eye	See instructions for administering eye drops.
Lodine	*Etodolac*	Pain, inflammation	See NSAID.
Lomefloxacin	Maxaquin	Antibiotic, infection	May cause an increased sensitivity of skin to the sun, sunburn occurs much more easily. Do not give with Carafate (sucralfate), antacids, zinc, or iron. See Ciprofloxacin.
Lomotil	*Diphenoxylate/atropine*	Diarrhea	May cause drowsiness, dizziness, dry mouth, constipation. Residents should avoid alcohol and use caution when taking other drugs that cause drowsiness.
Loperamide	Imodium	Diarrhea	See Imodium.
Lopid	*Gemfibrozil*	Lowers blood cholesterol	May cause stomach upset, abdominal pain, diarrhea, nausea, vomiting, fatigue. Give before meals.
Lopressor	*Metoprolol*	High blood pressure, angina	See Beta blockers.

Italic = generic name Red = brand name Boldface = drug class information

GENERIC AND BRAND NAME DRUGS		TREATMENT USES	CAREGIVER GUIDELINES
Lorazepam	Ativan	Anxiety, insomnia, seizures, agitation	See Benzodiazepines.
Lorelco	*Probucol*	Lowers blood cholesterol	May cause GI problems, headache. Give with meals.
Lortab	*Hydrocodone/APAP, Vicodin*	Pain relief	See Narcotic analgesics.
Lotensin	*Benazepril*	High blood pressure, congestive heart failure	See ACE inhibitors.
Lovastatin	Mevacor	Lowers blood cholesterol	May cause GI problems, headache. Give with meals.
Loxapine	Loxitane	Severe mental problems	See Antipsychotics.
Loxitane	*Loxapine*	Severe mental problems	See Antipsychotics.
Lozol	*Indapamide*	High blood pressure, edema, heart failure	See Diuretics.
Ludiomil	*Maprotiline*	Depression	See Tricyclic antidepressants.
Magaldrate	Riopan	Heartburn, stomach upset	May interfere with absorption of some antibiotics.
Magnesium hydroxide	Milk of Magnesia	Constipation	May cause diarrhea. Can interfere with absorption of many antibiotics.
Magnesium oxide	Mag-Ox	Heartburn, stomach upset	May cause diarrhea.
Magnesium trilisate	Gaviscon	Heartburn, stomach upset	May cause diarrhea or constipation.
Maxaquin	*Lomefloxacin*	Antibiotic, infection	See Cipirofloxicin. See Lomefloxacin.
Maxzide	*Triamterene/ hydrochlorothiazide*	High blood pressure, edema (swelling), CHF	See Diuretics.
Meclizine	Antivert	Motion sickness, vertigo	May cause drowsiness, restlessness, excitation, difficulty with urination, low blood pressure.
Mellaril	*Thioridazine*	Severe mental problems	See Antipsychotics.
Meperidine	Demerol	Pain relief	See Narcotic analgesics.

Generic and Brand Name Drugs		Treatment Uses	Caregiver Guidelines
Metaproterenol	Alupent	Chronic obstructive pulmonary disease (COPD), asthma	See Bronchodilators.
Metformin	Glucophage	Diabetes	See Glucophage.
Methocarbamol	Robaxin	Muscle relaxant	May cause drowsiness, slow heart rate, low blood pressure.
Methylcellulose	Citrucel	Laxative, constipation	Give with at least 8 oz of water or juice.
Methyldopa	Aldomet	High blood pressure	May cause low blood pressure, dizziness when standing up, sexual dysfunction, water retention, drowsiness, depression, headaches.
Methylphenidate	Ritalin	Central nervous system stimulant for narcolepsy, depression	May cause agitation, nervousness, confusion, headache, rapid heart rate, dizziness.
Metoclopramide	Reglan	Stomach acid reflux. Relieve symptoms of nausea, vomiting, heartburn	May cause irritability, confusion, drowsiness. Give before meals.
Metoprolol	Lopressor	High blood pressure, angina; also used for prevention of heart attack	See Beta blockers.
Mevacor	*Lovastatin*	Lowers blood cholesterol	May cause GI problems, headache. Give with meals.
Mexiletine	Mexitil	Irregular heartbeat, occasionally pain	May cause irregular heartbeat, dizziness, tremor, fever, sore throat, jaundice. Give with food.
Micatin	*Miconazole,* Monistat	Fungal infections (skin, vaginal)	Follow application instructions carefully.
Miconazole	Micatin, Monistat	Fungal infections	See Micatin.
Micro-K	*KCL, potassium chloride*	Potassium supplement	May cause nausea, vomiting, diarrhea, gas, abdominal discomfort. Liquid has bitter taste.
Micronase	DiaBeta, *Glyburide*	Diabetes	See Glipizide.

Italic = generic name   Red = brand name   Boldface = drug class information

GENERIC AND BRAND NAME DRUGS		TREATMENT USES	CAREGIVER GUIDELINES
Minocin	*Minocycline*	Antibiotic	See Demeclocycline.
Misoprostol	Cytotec	Prevents stomach ulcers from NSAID use	May cause headache, abdominal pain, gas, and diarrhea.
Moban	*Molindone*	Severe mental problems	See Antipsychotics.
Molindone	Moban	Severe mental problems	See Antipsychotics.
Monistat	Micatin, *Miconazole*	Fungal infections	See Micatin.
Monopril	*Fosinopril*	High blood pressure	See ACE inhibitors.
Morphine	MS Contin, Roxanol solution	Relief of severe pain	See Narcotic analgesics.
Motrin	*Ibuprofen*, Advil, many others	Pain, inflammation	Should be taken with food to reduce stomach irritation. See NSAID.
MS Contin	*Morphine*	Relief of severe pain	See Narcotic analgesics.
Mupirocin	Bactroban	Skin infection	May cause rash, burning, itching.
Mysoline	*Primidone*	Seizures (epilepsy)	May cause drowsiness, GI upset. Give with meals. Residents should avoid alcohol and use caution when taking other drugs that cause drowsiness.
Nabumetone	Relafen	Pain, inflammation	See NSAID.
Nadolol	Corgard	High blood pressure, angina ·	See Beta blockers.
Nafcillin	Nafcil, Unipen	Antibiotic, infection	See Amoxicillin.
Naphazoline	Privine, Vasocon, Naphcon, others	Spray: colds, nasal congestion. Eyedrops: minor irritation or redness	May cause rapid heart rate, loss of appetite, increased blood pressure. See instructions for administering eye drops.
Naprosyn	Aleve, *Naproxen*, Anaprox	Pain, inflammation	Should be taken with food to reduce stomach irritation. See NSAID.
Naproxen	Aleve, Naprosyn, Anaprox	Pain, inflammation	Should be taken with food to reduce stomach irritation. See NSAID.

GENERIC AND BRAND NAME DRUGS		TREATMENT USES	CAREGIVER GUIDELINES
Narcotic analgesics	*Codeine,* Darvocet-N, Darvon, Demerol, Dilaudid, Duragesic, *Fentanyl, Hydrocodone, Hydromorphone,* Lortab, *Meperidine, Morphine,* MS Contin, *Oxycodone,* Pentazocine, Percocet, *Propoxyphene,* Talwin, Tylox, Vicodin	Relief of moderate to severe pain	**Residents may require higher and higher doses if used regularly. May cause sedation, nausea, impaired breathing, constipation, blurry vision, and confusion. When dose is lowered significantly they can cause withdrawal symptoms of nervousness, nausea, rapid heartbeat, sweating, and abdominal cramping. The sedative effects of these drugs is increased if given with other sedating drugs or alcohol.**
Navane	*Thiothixene*	Severe mental problems	See Antipsychotics.
Nefazodone	Serzone	Antidepressant	See Fluoxetine.
Neomycin	Many combinations	Bacterial infections	Skin ointment or cream. Resident may develop an allergic skin reaction.
Neo-Synephrine	*Phenylephrine*	Glaucoma, red and irritated eyes, nasal congestion	May cause nervousness or rapid heart rate if used excessively. See instructions for administering eye drops and nose drops.
Nicardipine	Cardene	Angina, high blood pressure, congestive heart failure	See Calcium channel blockers.
Nifedipine	Adalat, Procardia	Angina, high blood pressure	See Calcium channel blockers.
Nitro-Bid, Nitrodisc, Nitro-Dur	*Nitroglycerin*	Angina	May cause headache, dizziness. See instructions for application of skin patch.
Nitroglycerin	Nitrostat-sublingual tablets, Nitrolingual spray	Angina	May cause headache, dizziness. Put tablet under tongue for relief in 5 to 10 minutes. Discard 6 months after opening. Store tightly closed; do not change containers. See instructions for sublingual tablets.
Nizatidine	Axid	Stomach and bowel ulcers, heartburn	See H-2 blockers.

Italic = generic name Red = brand name Boldface = drug class information

GENERIC AND BRAND NAME DRUGS		TREATMENT USES	CAREGIVER GUIDELINES
Noctec	*Chloral hydrate*	Insomnia	May cause excessive drowsiness, confusion, headache, nausea. May be habit forming. Residents should avoid alcohol and use caution when taking other sedating drugs.
Nolvadex	*Tamoxifen*	Prevention of breast cancer recurrence, as well as primary prevention	May cause vomiting, vaginal bleeding, or itching.
Norfloxacin	Chibroxin, Noroxin	Antibiotic	Do not give with Carafate (sucralfate), antacids, zinc, or iron. See Ciprofloxacin.
Normodyne	*Labetalol*	High blood pressure	See Beta blockers.
Noroxin	*Norfloxacin*	Antibiotic	See Ciprofloxacin.
Norpace	*Disopyramide*	Irregular heartbeat	May cause chest pains, nervousness, dizziness. See Anticholinergic drugs for additional side-effects.
Norpramin	*Desipramine*	Depression	See Tricyclic antidepressants.
Nortriptyline	Aventyl, Pamelor	Depression	See Tricyclic antidepressants.
NSAID (Nonsteroidal anti-inflammatory drugs)	Advil, Aleve, Ansaid, *Aspirin, Choline magnesium trisalicylate,* Daypro, *Diclofenac,* Disalcid, *Etodolac,* Feldene, *Flurbiprofen,* Ibuprofen, Indocin, *Indomethacin, Ketoprofen, Ketorolac,* Lodine, Motrin, *Nabumetone,* Naprosyn, *Naproxen,* Orudis, *Oxaprozin, Piroxicam, Profenal,* Relafen, Salsalate, *Suprofen,* Tolectin, *Tolmetin,* Toradol, Trilisate, Voltaren	**Pain relief and inflammation**	**May cause bleeding from ulcers in the stomach or bowel, nausea, diarrhea, constipation, abdominal discomfort, upset stomach, gas, loss of appetite, ringing in the ears, swelling of the ankles. Do not give nonprescription NSAIDs to residents with aspirin sensitivity without consulting the doctor. There is rarely a reason to give more than one of these drugs at a time—if more than one is prescribed or if a nonprescription NSAID is being used as well as a prescription one, discuss with a doctor. Give with food to reduce stomach discomfort.**

Generic and Brand Name Drugs		Treatment Uses	Caregiver Guidelines
Ocufen	*Flurbiprofen*	Reduces eye inflammation	See instructions for administering eye drops.
Ocupress	*Cartelol*	Glaucoma	See instructions for administering eye drops.
Ocusert-Pilo	*Pilocarpine*	Glaucoma	Special sacs are placed in the eye for 7 days.
Ofloxacin	Floxin, Ocuflox (eye)	Antibiotic, infection	Do not give with Carafate (sucralfate), antacids, zinc, or iron. See Ciprofloxacin.
Omeprazole	Prilosec	See Prevacid	See Prevacid.
Orinase	*Tolbutamide*	Diabetes	May cause low blood sugar. See Glipizide.
Orudis	*Ketoprofen*	Pain, inflammation	See NSAID.
Oxacillin	Bactocill, Prostaphlin	Antibiotic	See Amoxicillin.
Oxaprozin	Daypro	Pain, arthritis	See NSAID.
Oxybutynin	Ditropan	Urinary spasms	See Anticholinergic drugs.
Oxycodone	Percocet (with Acetaminophen)	Pain, arthritis	See NSAID.
Oxymetazoline	Afrin, others	Colds, nasal congestion	May cause rapid heart rate, loss of appetite, increased blood pressure.
Oxytriphylline	Choledyl	Increases air to lungs	See Theophylline.
Pamelor	Aventyl, *Nortriptyline*	Depression	See Tricyclic antidepressants.
Pancrelipase	Pancrease, others	Poor digestion	Do not crush tablets.
Parafon Forte	*Chlorzoxazone*	Muscle relaxant	May cause dizziness, urine may turn orange or purple. Residents should avoid alcohol and use caution when taking other drugs that cause drowsiness. Give with food or milk.

Italic = generic name   Red = brand name   Boldface = drug class information

GENERIC AND BRAND NAME DRUGS		TREATMENT USES	CAREGIVER GUIDELINES
Parlodel	*Bromocriptine*	Parkinson's disease	May cause nausea and drowsiness at beginning of therapy, low blood pressure, dizziness, nightmares, insomnia, hallucinations. Residents should avoid alcohol and use caution when taking other drugs that cause drowsiness. Give with food or milk.
Paroxetine	Paxil	Antidepressant	See Prozac.
Paxil	*Paroxetine*	Antidepressant	See Prozac.
Paxipam	*Halazepam*	Anxiety, agitation	See Benzodiazepines.
Penetrex	*Enoxacin*	Antibiotic	See Ciprofloxacin.
Penicillin G, VK	Many combinations	Antibiotic	See Amoxicillin.
Pentazocine	Talwin (and NX)	Pain relief	May cause headache. See Narcotic analgesics.
Pentoxifylline	Trental	Improves blood flow to arms, legs	May cause dizziness, headache, change in heart rate.
Pepcid	*Famotidine*	Stomach and bowel ulcers, heartburn	See H-2 blockers.
Percocet	*Oxycodone/APAP*	Pain relief	See Narcotic analgesics, APAP.
Periactin	*Cyproheptadine*	Allergies, appetite stimulation	See Anticholinergic and Antihistamine drugs.
Perphenazine	Trilafon	Severe mental problems	See Antipsychotics.
Persantine	*Dipyridamole*	Prevents blood clots, increases blood flow to the heart.	May cause dizziness, flushing, increased bruising or bleeding.
Phenazopyridine	Pyridium	Urinary pain	Turns urine red or orange; may stain clothing. Give after meals.
Phenergan	*Promethazine*	Allergies, cough, nausea, vomiting, insomnia	See Anticholinergic drugs and Antihistamines.
Phenobarbital	Luminal	Seizures (epilepsy)	May cause drowsiness. Residents should avoid alcohol and use caution when taking other drugs that cause drowsiness.

GENERIC AND BRAND NAME DRUGS		TREATMENT USES	CAREGIVER GUIDELINES
Phenylephrine (eye)	Isopto Frin, others	Eye redness due to irritation	May cause nervousness or rapid heart rate if used excessively. See instructions for administering eye drops.
Phenylephrine (nasal)	Neo-Synephrine	Colds, nasal congestion	May cause fast heart rate, loss of appetite, increased blood pressure. See instructions for administering nose drops.
Phenylpropa- nolamine	Many combinations	Nasal congestion, appetite suppression	May cause rapid heart rate, loss of appetite, increased blood pressure.
Phenytoin	Dilantin	Seizures (epilepsy)	May cause drowsiness, vision problems, unsteadiness, marked drowsiness.
Phospholine Iodide	Echothiophate	Glaucoma	See instructions for administering eye drops.
Physostigmine	Eserine	Glaucoma	See instructions for administering eye drops.
Pilocarpine	Many combinations	Glaucoma	See instructions for administering eye drops.
Pindolol	Visken	High blood pressure	See Beta blockers.
Piroxicam	Feldene	Inflammation, pain	See NSAID.
Plendil	*Felodipine*	High blood pressure	See Calcium channel blockers.
Polycillin	*Ampicillin*	Antibiotic, infection	See Amoxicillin.
Polymyxin B	Many combinations	Antibiotic, skin infections	Can cause allergic rash.
Pramoxine	Many combinations	Hemorrhoids, reduces pain and itching	Local anesthetic. Causes numbness
Pravachol	*Pravastatin*	Lowers blood cholesterol	May cause GI problems, headache. Give with meals.
Prednisone	Deltasone	Inflammation, severe COPD, arthritis	Give with meals. May cause GI ulcers, weakness, confusion, insomnia, weight gain, personality change. Can cause or worsen diabetes. If resident has been taking for a long time, do not stop abruptly—contact the doctor if resident refuses medication.

Italic = generic name Red = brand name Boldface = drug class information

GENERIC AND BRAND NAME DRUGS		TREATMENT USES	CAREGIVER GUIDELINES
Premarin	*Conjugated estrogens*	Replacement therapy, prevention of osteoporosis	May cause sudden severe headache, vomiting, visual or speech disturbance, shortness of breath, chest pain, depression, unusual bleeding.
Prevacid	*Lansoprazole*	Conditions caused by excessive stomach acid such as ulcers or damage to the esophagus	May cause abdominal pain, diarrhea. Give before meals. Do not open, chew, or crush capsule. Be sure doctor knows any other drugs resident is taking.
Prilosec	*Omeprazole*	See Prevacid	See Prevacid.
Primidone	Mysoline	Seizures (epilepsy)	See Mysoline.
Prinivil	*Lisinopril,* Zestril	High blood pressure, congestive heart failure	See ACE inhibitors.
Pro-Banthine	*Propantheline*	GI spasms	See Anticholinergic drugs.
Probenecid	Benemid	Gouty arthritis	See Benemid.
Probucol	Lorelco	Lowers blood cholesterol	May cause GI problems, headache. Give with meals.
Procainamide	Procan, Procan SR, Pronestyl	Irregular heartbeat	May cause irregular heartbeat, sores in mouth, throat, gums, fever, confusion, hallucinations, delusions.
Procardia	Adalat, Adalat CC, *Nifedipine*	Angina, high blood pressure	Give Adalat CC on empty stomach. See Calcium channel blockers.
Prochlorperazine	Compazine	Nausea, vomiting	See Antipsychotics.
Profenal	*Suprofen*	Reduces inflammation	See NSAID.
Prolixin	*Fluphenazine*	Severe mental problems	See Antipsychotics.
Promazine	Sparine	Severe mental problems	See Antipsychotics.
Promethazine	Phenergan	Allergies, cough, nausea, vomiting, insomnia	See Anticholinergic drugs and Antihistamines.
Pronestyl	*Procainamide*	Irregular heartbeat	See Procainamide.
Propafenone	Rythmol	Irregular heartbeat	May cause palpitations, chest pain, difficulty breathing, blurred vision, fever, sore throat, bleeding, bruising.

GENERIC AND BRAND NAME DRUGS		TREATMENT USES	CAREGIVER GUIDELINES
Propantheline	Pro-Banthine	Bowel and stomach spasms	See Anticholinergic drugs.
Propoxyphene	Darvon	Pain relief	See Narcotic analgesics.
Propoxyphene N with APAP	Darvocet-N	Pain relief	See Narcotic analgesics.
Propranolol	Inderal	High blood pressure, angina, irregular heart-beat, tremors	See Beta blockers.
Proscar	*Finasteride*	Prostrate enlargement	See Finasteride
ProSom	*Estazolam*	Insomnia	See Benzodiazepines.
Prostaphlin	*Oxacillin*	Antibiotic	See Amoxicillin.
Proventil	*Albuterol,* Ventolin	Asthma, chronic obstruc-tive pulmonary disease (COPD)	See Bronchodilators.
Prozac	*Fluoxetine*	Depression, obsessive–compulsive disorder	May cause anxiety, nervousness, hyperactivity, insomnia, loss of appetite, headache, nausea, diarrhea, weakness, drowsiness, tremor, sweat-ing, sexual problems.
Pseudoephedrine	Sudafed	Nasal congestion	May cause nervousness and excitabil-ity. May increase blood pressure.
Pyridium	*Phenazopyridine*	Urinary pain, bladder spasms	Turns urine red or orange; may stain clothing. Give after meals.
Questran	*Cholestyramine*	Lowers blood cholesterol	See Cholestyramine
Quinapril	Accupril	High blood pressure, congestive heart failure	See ACE inhibitors.
Quinidex	*Quinidine* (sustained release)	Irregular heartbeat	May cause irregular heartbeat, confu-sion, disorientation, dementia, impaired hearing or vision, bleeding or bruising, fever, diarrhea.
Quinidine	Quinidex	Irregular heartbeat	See Quinidex
Quinine	Quinamm	Leg cramps	May cause headache, ringing in the ears, nausea, irregular heartbeat.

Italic = generic name Red = brand name Boldface = drug class information

GENERIC AND BRAND NAME DRUGS		TREATMENT USES	CAREGIVER GUIDELINES
Ramipril	Altace	High blood pressure, congestive heart failure	See ACE inhibitors.
Ranitidine	Zantac	Stomach and bowel ulcers, heartburn	See H-2 blockers.
Reglan	*Metoclopramide*	Stomach acid reflux, nausea	May cause irritability, confusion, drowsiness. Give before meals.
Relafen	*Nabumetone*	Pain, inflammation	See NSAID.
Restoril	*Temazepam*	Insomnia	Give one hour before bedtime. Encourage resident not to use every night. See Estazolam and Benzodiazephines.
Risperdal	*Risperidone*	Severe mental problems	See Antipsychotics.
Ritalin	*Methylphenidate*	Central nervous system stimulant for narcolepsy, depression	May cause agitation, nervousness, confusion, headache, rapid heart rate, dizziness.
Robaxin	*Methocarbamol*	Muscle relaxant	May cause drowsiness, slow heart rate, low blood pressure.
Rythmol	*Propafenone*	Irregular heartbeat	May cause palpitations, chest pain, difficulty breathing, blurred vision, fever, sore throat, bleeding, bruising.
Salsalate	Disalcid	Pain, inflammation	See NSAID.
Scopolamine (eye)	*Hyoscine*	Glaucoma	See instructions for administering eye drops. See Anticholinergic drugs.
Sectral	*Acebutolol*	Irregular heartbeat, hypertension, angina	See Beta blockers.
Seldane, Seldane-D	*Terfenadine* with and without decongestant	Allergies, bronchial spasms	There are many possible drug interactions. Be sure the doctor is aware of all other medications the resident is taking. See Pseudoephedrine.
Selegiline	Eldepryl	Parkinson's disease	May cause dizziness, severe headache, hallucinations, depression, insomnia, involuntary movements, irregular heart beat.

GENERIC AND BRAND NAME DRUGS		TREATMENT USES	CAREGIVER GUIDELINES
Septra, Septra DS	Bactrim, Bactrim DS, *Trimethoprim/sulpha-methoxazole*	Antibiotic, infections	May cause rash. Encourage fluid intake.
Sertraline	Zoloft	Depression	See Fluoxetine.
Serzone	*Nefazodone*	Antidepressant	See Prozac.
Simethicone	Mylicon	Relieves cramping and bloating from gas	Often given with antacids.
Simvastatin	Zocor	Lowers blood cholesterol	See Fluvastatin.
Sinemet, Sinemet CR	*Levodopa/carbidopa*	Parkinson's disease	May cause anxiety, insomnia, nervousness, hallucinations, fast or fluttering heartbeat, low blood pressure when standing up; increase risk of falls. Give on empty stomach unless stomach problems.
Sinequan	Adapin, *Doxepin*	Depression, anxiety	See Tricyclic antidepressants.
Slo-bid	*Theophylline*	Increases air to lungs	May cause nausea, vomiting, insomnia, palpitations, nervousness, irritability. Resident should avoid taking large amounts of beverages containing caffeine (coffee, tea, some sodas).
Sodium phosphate	Fleets enema	Constipation	Saline enema. See instructions on administering enemas.
Sodium sulfacetamide	Bleth-10, Sulamyd	Eye infections	May sensitize eye to bright light. See instructions for administering eye drops.
Sorbitrate	*Isosorbide dinitrate,* Isordil	Angina, congestive heart failure, esophagus spasm	May cause dizziness increasing the risk of falls when standing up after sitting; also may cause headache, rapid heartbeat, flushing.
Sparine	*Promazine*	Severe mental problems	See Antipsychotics.
Spectrobid	*Bacampicillin*	Antibiotic	See Amoxicillin.
Sucralfate	Carafate	Stomach and bowel ulcers	See Carafate.

Italic = generic name   Red = brand name   Boldface = drug class information

Generic and Brand Name Drugs		Treatment Uses	Caregiver Guidelines
Sudafed	*Pseudoephedrine*	Colds, nasal congestion	May cause nervousness and excitability. Caution with residents being treated for high blood pressure.
Sulamyd	*Sulfacetamide*	Eye infections	See Sodium Sulfacetamide.
Sulfisoxazole	Gantrisin	Antibiotic	May cause rash. Give with 8 oz of liquids
Suprax	*Cefixime*	Antibiotic	Allergic reaction may occur in residents with penicillin allergy. See Amoxicillin.
Suprofen	Profenal	Arthritis, pain relief	See NSAID. See instructions for administering eye drops.
Symmetrel	*Amantadine*	Parkinson's disease, influenza (flu)	May cause dizziness, headache, loss of appetite, nervousness, irritability, difficulty sleeping, blurred vision, urination problems, confusion, mental changes.
Synthroid	Levothroid, *Levothyroxine*	Thyroid replacement therapy	May cause chest pain, weight loss, nervousness, fast heartbeat, sweating, insomnia.
Tagamet	*Cimetidine*	Stomach and bowel ulcers, heartburn	See H-2 blockers.
Talwin (and NX)	*Pentazocine*	Pain relief	May cause headache. See Narcotic analgesics.
Tambocor	*Flecainide*	Irregular heartbeat	May cause irregular heartbeat, dizziness, fatigue, tremor, nervousness, headache.
Tamoxifen	Nolvadex	Prevention of breast cancer recurrence, as well as primary prevention	May cause vomiting, vaginal bleeding, or itching.
Tegopen	*Cloxacillin*	Antibiotic	See Amoxicillin.
Tegretol	*Carbamazepine*	Seizures, facial pain	May cause increased sensitivity to sun. Report vision or eye movement problems, unusual bleeding or bruising, light colored stools, drowsiness, dizziness, mouth sores promptly to doctor.

Drugs, Generic and Brand Names		Treatment Uses	Caregiver Guidelines
Temazepam	Restoril	Insomnia	Give one hour before bedtime. Avoid nightly use. See Benzodiazepines.
Tenex	*Guanfacine*	High blood pressure	May cause dizziness, drowsiness, headache. Give at bedtime.
Tenormin	*Atenolol,* others	Angina, high blood pressure, irregular heartbeat, prevention of recurrent heart attack	See Beta blockers.
Terazosin	Hytrin	High blood pressure, prostate enlargement	May cause low blood pressure, dizziness and fainting when getting up, especially with first dose.
Terfenadine	Seldane, Seldane-D	Allergies, decongestant	See Seldane. See Pseudoephedrine.
Tetracycline	Achromycin, many others	Antibiotic, infection	Do not give with antacids or dairy products. Give 1 hour before or 2 hours after meals. May cause rash, nausea, diarrhea, dizziness, increased sensitivity to the sun.
Tetrahydrozoline (nasal)	Tyzine, others	Colds, nasal congestion	Overuse can result in congestion. May cause rapid heart rate, loss of appetite, increased blood pressure.
Theo-Dur	*Theophylline*	Increases air to lungs, opens airways	See Theophylline.
Theophylline	Elixophyllin, Slo-bid, Theo-Dur, Uniphyl	Increases air to lungs opens airways	May cause nausea, vomiting, insomnia, palpitations, nervousness, irritability. Resident should avoid taking large amounts of beverages containing caffeine (coffee, tea, some sodas).
Thioridazine	Mellaril	Severe mental problems	See Antipsychotics.
Thiothixene	Navane	Severe mental problems	See Antipsychotics.
Thorazine	*Chlorpromazine*	Severe mental problems	See Antipsychotics.
Ticlid	*Ticlopidine*	Blood clot and prevention of stroke	May cause unusual bleeding, fevers, chills, sore throat.
Tigan	*Trimethobenzamide*	Nausea and vomiting	May cause drowsiness.

Italic = generic name Red = brand name Boldface = drug class information

Generic and Brand Name Drugs		Treatment Uses	Caregiver Guidelines
Timolol	Blocarden	Hypertension, recurrent heart attack, prevention of migraine	See Beta blockers.
Timoptic	*Timolol*	Glaucoma	See instructions for administering eye drops. See Atenolol.
Tindal	*Acetophenazine*	Severe mental problems	See Antipsychotics.
Tobramycin	Tobrex	Eye infection	See instructions for administering eye drops.
Tocainide	Tonocard	Irregular heartbeat	May cause fast or slow heart rate, unusual bleeding, bruising, sore throat, fever, chills, breathing difficulties, drowsiness. Give with food.
Tofranil	*Imipramine*	Depression	See Tricyclic antidepressants.
Tolazamide	Tolinase	Diabetes	See Glipizide.
Tolbutamide	Orinase	Diabetes	See Glipizide
Tolectin	*Tolmetin*	Pain, inflammation	See NSAID.
Tolinase	*Tolazamide*	Diabetes	See Glipizide.
Tolmetin	Tolectin	Pain, inflammation	See NSAID.
Tonocard	*Tocainide*	Irregular heartbeat	See Tocainide.
Toradol	*Ketorolac*	Pain, inflammation	See NSAID.
Tramadol	Ultram	Pain relief	May cause dizziness, constipation, sleepiness, nausea, confusion, headache. Residents should avoid alcohol.
Tranxene	*Clorazepate*	Anxiety	See Benzodiazepines.
Trazodone	Desyrel	Depression, insomnia; aggressive behavior, panic disorders	See Tricyclic antidepressants.
Trental	*Pentoxifylline*	Improves blood flow to arms, legs	May cause dizziness, headache, heart rate changes. Give with meals.

GENERIC AND BRAND NAME DRUGS		TREATMENT USES	CAREGIVER GUIDELINES
Triamterene/ hydrochlorothiazide	Dyazide, Maxzide	High blood pressure, edema (swelling)	See Diuretics.
Triavil	*Perphenazine, Amitriptyline*	Severe mental problems	See Antipsychotics and Antidepressants.
Triazolam	Halcion	Insomnia	May cause loss of memory of recent events. See Benzodiazepines.
Tricyclic antidepressants	Adapin, *Amitriptyline, Amoxapine,* Asendin, Aventyl, *Desipramine,* Desyrel, Doxepin, Elavil, *Imipramine,* Ludiomil, *Maprotiline,* Norpramin, *Nortriptyline,* Pamelor, *Sinequan,* Tofranil, *Trazadone*	**Depression, pain from nerve damage, especially in diabetics and from "pinched nerves"**	**May cause dizziness, low blood pressure, confusion, fast or irregular heartbeat, nervousness, agitation. Residents should avoid alcohol and use caution when taking other drugs that cause drowsiness.**
Trifluridine	Viroptic	Viral eye infections, herpes infections	See instructions for administering eye drops.
Trihexyphenidyl	Artane	Parkinson's disease	See Anticholinergics.
Trilafon	*Perphenazine*	Severe mental problems	See Antipsychotics.
Trimethoben- zamide	Tigan	Nausea and vomiting	May cause drowsiness.
Trimethoprim/ sulfa- methoxazole	Bactrim, Bactrim DS, Septra, Septra DS, TMP-SMZ	Antibiotic, infection	May cause rash. Encourage fluid intake.
Tylenol with codeine	*Acetaminophen (APAP) and codeine,* Tylenol #2, #3, and #4	Relief of moderate to severe pain Pain relief	See Narcotic analgesics.
Ultracef	*Cefadroxil,* Duricef	Antibiotic, infection	See Amoxicillin.
Ultram	*Tramadol*	Pain relief	May cause constipation, sleepiness, nausea, confusion.

Italic = generic name Red = brand name Boldface = drug class information

GENERIC AND BRAND NAME DRUGS		TREATMENT USES	CAREGIVER GUIDELINES
Unipen	Nafcil, *Nafcillin*	Antibiotic	See Amoxicillin.
Uniphyl	*Theophylline*	Increases air to lungs, opens airways	See Theophylline.
Urecholine	*Bethanechol*	Excessive urinary retention in bladder	May cause nausea, vomiting, diarrhea, abdominal cramps, flushing, dizziness. Give 1 hour before or 2 hours after meals.
Urispas	*Flavoxate*	To relieve urinary bladder spasms that cause incontinence	See Anticholinergic drugs.
Valium	*Diazepam*	Anxiety, agitation, muscle relaxant, seizures	Use caution when giving medication to elderly residents due to long-lasting effects and the possibility of falls. See Benzodiazepines.
Valproic acid	Depakene	Seizures (epilepsy); behavior modification in selected cases	May cause drowsiness, tremor, unsteadiness, confusion, restlessness, dizziness, sore throat, fever, fatigue. Give with food or milk. Do not break or crush tablets. Do not give with carbonated beverages.
Vancocin	*Vancomycin*	Antibiotic	Can damage hearing and cause ringing in the ears—contact doctor immediately if these develop.
Vancomycin	Vancocin, Vancoled	Antibiotic, infection	See Vancocin.
Vantin	*Cefpodoxime*	Antibiotic, infection	See Amoxicillin.
Vascor	*Bepridil*	Angina	See Calcium channel blockers.
Vasotec	*Enalapril*	High blood pressure, congestive heart failure	See ACE inhibitors.
Velosef	Anspor, *Cephradine*	Antibiotic, infection	See Amoxicillin.
Venlafaxine	Effexor	Depression	May cause insomnia, dizziness, nervousness, loss of appetite, sexual dysfunction in men, drowsiness, increased blood pressure. Resident should avoid alcohol. Notify doctor of all other medications resident is taking.

GENERIC AND BRAND NAME DRUGS		TREATMENT USES	CAREGIVER GUIDELINES
Ventolin	*Albuterol,* Proventil	Asthma, chronic obstructive pulmonary disease (COPD)	See Bronchodilators.
Verapamil	Calan, Calan SR, Isoptin, Isoptin SR	High blood pressure, angina, irregular heartbeat	May cause constipation. See Calcium channel blockers.
Vibramycin	Doryx, *Doxycycline*	Antibiotic	See Tetracycline.
Vicodin	*Hydrocodone/APAP,* Lortab	Relief of moderate to severe pain	See Narcotic analgesics.
Vira-A	*Vidarabine*	Herpes infections of eye	See instructions for administering eye drops.
Viroptic	*Trifluridine*	Herpes infections of eye	See instructions for administering eye drops.
Visken	*Pindolol*	High blood pressure	See Beta blockers.
Vistaril	Atarax, *Hydroxyzine*	Itching, anxiety, sedation	See Antihistamines and Anticholinergic drugs.
Voltaren	*Diclofenac*	Pain, inflammation	See NSAID.
Warfarin	Coumadin	Anticoagulant (blood thinner)	Call doctor immediately if resident develops unusual bleeding or bruising. Notify other doctors of all other medications resident is taking.
Wellbutrin	*Bupropion*	Depression	May cause weight loss, dizziness, confusion, insomnia, restlessness, anxiety, agitation. Residents should avoid alcohol and use caution when taking other drugs that cause drowsiness.
Xanax	*Alprazolam*	Anxiety, agitation, panic disorder, sometimes insomnia	See Benzodiazepines.
Xylometazoline	Otrivin	Nasal congestion	Overuse can result in congestion. May cause fast heart rate, loss of appetite, increased blood pressure.
Zantac	*Ranitidine*	Stomach and bowel ulcers, heartburn	See H-2 blockers.

Italic = generic name   Red = brand name   Boldface = drug class information

Drugs, Generic and Brand Names		Treatment Uses	Caregiver Guidelines
Zestril	*Lisinopril,* Prinivil	High blood pressure, congestive heart failure	See ACE inhibitors.
Zinacef	Ceftin, *Cefuroxime,*	Antibiotic	See Amoxicillin.
Zithromax	*Azithromycin*	Antibiotic	Should not be given with antacids. See Clarithromycin.
Zocor	*Simvastatin*	Lowers blood cholesterol	See Fluvastatin.
Zoloft	*Sertraline*	Depression	See Prozac.
Zolpidem	Ambien	Insomnia	May cause headache, daytime drowsiness, memory loss. Residents should avoid alcohol and use caution when taking other drugs that cause drowsiness.
Zyloprim	*Allopurinol*	Gouty arthritis	May cause drowsiness, chills, fever, joint or muscle pain, sore throat, nausea, vomiting, skin rash. Do not give vitamin C without doctor OK.

Appendix 1
Residential Care Facility Health Resources

There are essentially two kinds of resources available to RCF managers and caregivers—those that are designed to help you operate and meet your resident's needs in an effective manner and those that are designed to help people with specific kinds of diseases or problems. Because social and activities services play such an important part in providing for the needs of elderly people, some resources directed at those services are included.

Most services for the elderly are community based; some have a government connection, but most others are sponsored by non-profit groups and organizations. Always check your phone book for information on these groups. Usually you need only identify one key organization to obtain information on all similar resources in the community.

National Resources for General Information

Administration on Aging
Office of the Secretary
U.S. Department of Health and Human Services
330 Independence Avenue SW
Washington, DC 20402
(202) 619–0724
Publishes *The Aging Network* lists of programs and services.

American Association of Retired Persons
601 E Street NW
Washington, DC 20049
Offers a wide variety of information and both free and fee-based services, although those related specifically to assisted living or RCFs are limited.

American Association of Homes and Services for the Aging
901 E Street NW, Suite 500
Washington, DC 20004-2837
(202) 783–2242
Advocate for non-profit assisted living/residential care facilities. Free consumer brochures; other publications, information with membership.

American Health Care Association
1201 L Street NW
Washington, DC 20005-4014
(202) 842–4444
Advocate for facilities providing all ranges of services from free-standing sub-acute care to skilled nursing and all levels of assisted living. Primarily for-profit membership, but includes non-profit members also.

American Society on Aging
833 Market Street, Suite 511
San Francisco, CA 94103-1824
(800) 537–9728
Composed of a variety of professionals, educators, and advocates.

National Association of Area Agencies on Aging
1112 16th Street NW, Suite 100
Washington, DC 20036
(202) 296–8130
Represents hundreds of mandated area agencies. Funds "Eldercare Locator" (see below). Particularly useful when there is no local clearinghouse organization to coordinate referral needs and information.

National Council on the Aging
409 Third Street SW
Washington, DC 20024
(202) 479–1200
Like the American Society on Aging, this is an umbrella group of different professionals and separate organizations involved in aging research and services.

National Institute on Aging
Public Information Office
Building 31, Rm 5C27
31 Center Drive
MSC 2292
Bethesda, MD 20892-2292
(301) 496–1752
Part of the National Institutes of Health (NIH); conducts extensive research, but also publishes free pamphlets intended for elderly persons.

Assisted Living for the Aged and Frail—Innovations in Design, Management, and Financing
Regnier, et. al.; Columbia University Press

Assisted Living in the US: A New Paradigm for Residential Care for Frail Older Persons?
Kane, Rosalie; American Association of Retired Persons
137 pg

The Caregiver's Guide
Caroline Rob, RN; Houghton Mifflin Company, Boston
1991, 458 pg,
A comprehensive look at health and safety provisions involved in caring for frail elderly persons. Designed primarily for individuals caring for elderly at home, but most of the information and principles apply to RCFs.

Choice, Challenge, and Companionship
Beverly Foundation, 1986
Includes instructions on creating a community resources guide.

Eldercare Locator
(800) 677–1116
A clearinghouse service that provides information on resources available in the field of aging throughout the country.

Guide to Housing Alternatives for Older Citizens
Consumer Report Books, 1985
Covers all levels of long-term housing and care from a consumer's perspective.

Handbook of Gerontological Services
A. Monk; Van Nostrand Reinhold Publishers
688 pg

Housing for the Aged
Regnier, Pynoos; Elsevier Science Publishing Company, 1987
Covers some operational aspects in addition to building concerns.

Residential Care for the Elderly
Baggett; Greenwood Press, 1989

Social and Medical Services in Housing for the Aged
National Institutes of Mental Health
U.S. Department of Health and Human Services

Working with the Elderly
Deichman, Kociecki; Prometheus Books, 1989

Resources for Specific Diseases

Alzheimer's Association
(800) 272–3900

American Cancer Society
1599 Clifton Road NE
Atlanta, GA 30329
(800) 227–2345
This well-known society offers programs, information, and literature. Local offices in many cities and towns.

Arthritis Foundation
P.O. Box 1900
Atlanta, GA 30326
(800) 283–7800
Provides free brochures, information. Many local offices available.

American Diabetes Association
1660 Duke Street
Alexandria, VA 22314
(800) 232–3472
Provides free brochures, information. Many local chapters.

American Speech-Language-Hearing Association
10801 Rockville Pike
Rockville, MD 20852
(800) 638–8255
Provides brochures, information on hearing and speech difficulties, sources for treatment.

American Heart Association
7272 Greenville Avenue
Dallas, TX 75231
(214) 373–6300
Many local affiliates offer programs, brochures, information.

National Diabetes Information Clearinghouse
1 Information Way
Bethesda, MD 20892-3560
(301) 654–3327

National Rehabilitation Information Center
8455 Colesville Road, Suite 935
Silver Spring, MD 20910-3319
(800) 346–2742
A clearinghouse of information established by the U.S. Department of Education.

National Stroke Association
8480 East Orchard Road, Suite 1000
Englewood, CO 80111-5015
(303) 771–1700
Provides information, publications, brochures; many local "Stroke Clubs."

APPENDIX 2

Measurement Equivalents

LIQUID MEASURES

HOUSEHOLD		APOTHECARY
1 teaspoon	=	60 drops
1 tablespoon	=	3 teaspoons
2 tablespoons	=	1 ounce
1 cup	=	8 ounces
2 cups	=	1 pint
1 pint	=	16 ounces
2 pints	=	1 quart
1 quart	=	32 ounces

METRIC MEASURES

1 cc is the same as 1 ml		
5 cc	=	1 teaspoon
15 cc	=	1 tablespoon
30 cc	=	1 ounce
240 cc	=	1 cup
480 cc	=	1 pint
960 cc	=	1 quart

APPENDIX 3

Common Medical Abbreviations

a	before	ECG, EKG	electrocardiogram, electrocardiograph	min	minute
ac	before meals			ml	milliliter
AD	right ear	EEG	electroencephalo-gram	MOM	milk of magnesia
AS	left ear			MS	morphine sulfate
AU	both ears	F	Fahrenheit	Na	sodium
ad lib	as desired	Fe	iron	no	number
APAP	acetaminophen	FeSO$_4$	ferrous sulfate	noct	night
ASA	aspirin	FSBG	finger stick blood glucose	NPO	nothing by mouth
aq	water			NS	normal saline
BID	twice a day	FSBS	finger stick blood sugar	NTG	nitroglycerin
BP	blood pressure	gm, g, Gm	gram	OD	right eye
c̄	with	GI	gastrointestinal	OS	left eye
C	Centigrade, Celcius	gtt	drop	OU	in each eye
Ca	calcium	h, hr	hour	OTC	over the counter
CA	cancer	HC	hydrocortisone	oz	ounce
cap	capsule	HCTZ	hydrochlorothi-azide	pc	after meals
cardiac	pertaining to the heart			per	through, or by
		HR	heart rate	po	by mouth
cl	chloride	hs	bedtime, hour of sleep	PR	by rectum
cc	cubic centimeter			prn	as needed, if necessary
CHF	congestive heart failure	IM	intramuscular		
		IV	intravenous	pt	pint
cm	centimeter	K	potassium	Pt	patient
CNS	central nervous system	KCl	potassium chloride	PT	physical therapy
		K, kg	kilogram	q	every, each
COPD	chronic obstructive pulmonary disease	L	liter	qd	every day
		LE	left eye	qh	every hour
CVA	cerebral vascular accident	mcg, μg	microgram	q2h	every two hours
		med	medication	q3h	every three hours
d	day	mEq	milliequivalent	qhs	every night
DC	discontinue	mg	milligram	qid	four times a day
dil	dilute				

continued on the following page

Common Medical Abbreviations continued

q noc	every night	sol	solution	URI	upper respiratory infection
qod	every other day	stat	immediately		
qow	every other week	subq	subcutaneous (between skin and muscle)	UTI	urinary tract infection
qt	quart			via	by way of
qw	every week	supp	suppository	VS	vital signs (TPR)
R	rectal	susp	suspension	wk	week
rep	repeat	syr	syrup	wt	weight
resp	respiration	tab	tablet		
RDA	Recommended Dietary Allowance	tid	three times a day		
Rx	prescription only, by prescription	tbsp, T	tablespoon		
		temp	temperature		
$\bar{s}$	without	TPR	temperature, pulse, respiration		
$\bar{ss}$	one half	troch	lozenges		
SC	subcutaneous (between skin and muscle)	tsp, t	teaspoon		
		U	units		
SL	sublingual (under the tongue)	ung	ointment		

APPENDIX 4
Drug References

*The following references are selected primarily based on their availability in book stores and ease of use for laypersons. There are many other quality references for health professionals that are very difficult for others to use. The references listed here will provide more than enough information for the RCF caregiver or manager. We suggest that you thumb through any reference before purchase to see if you are comfortable with the print size and book size and the way information is presented. Remember that the information provided is very conservative; that is, the authors tend to go overboard on cautions. Never change therapy, except in an emergency (e.g., a drug allergy), without consulting the resident's doctor. The publications listed range in price from approximately $5.00 to $30.00. Pictures of tablets and capsules do not include generics. Books that list drugs alphabetically by brand and generic name are usually easier for the average person to use than those that group drugs by therapeutic category and require frequent use of the index; books that provide special information on the use of medications in the elderly have extra value. Books more than 3 to 4 years old will not include a significant number of newer drugs. This is **not** intended to be a comprehensive listing.*

A Consumer's Dictionary of Medicines
Ruth Winter
Crown Trade Publications, 1993, 507 pages
General information only on a wide variety of drugs. Not a good primary reference.

AARP Pharmacy Service Prescription Drug Handbook
AARP, 1992, 1137 pages
Full sized reference with large print. Some pictures of drugs. Disease-based: must use index. Extra information about diseases. Good information on drug use, storage, and implications for elderly.

The ABCs of Prescription Drugs
Edward Edelson
Ivy Press, 1987, 1400 listings
Look for newer revision. Arranged by diseases or condition with alphabetized index available. Includes information on elderly. A bargain, but with significant limitations.

HOW TO SELECT A DRUG REFERENCE

Book design: durable hardcover vs paperback, page size, print size.

Information format: alphabetical vs therapeutic listings, brand vs generic name, illustrations.

Readability: Is it easy for you to understand?

Information provided: Good references should give you information on:

- What the drug does
- How to store the medication
- Precautions on use
- How to take the medication
- Food and drug interactions
- Side-effects that you can observe
- Missed dose, overdose, usual dose
- Special information on elderly use
- Tablet and capsule identification (not as important as other information)

About Your Medicines, 6th edition
USPC, 1991, 1046 pages
Similar in format to Consumer Reports published version, but paperback book size. Authoritative reference from the USPC (United States Pharmacopeial Convention, Inc.), with good emphasis on likely frequency as well as severity of side-effects. Newer drugs not included until new edition available. Combined therapeutic and generic name listing will require use of index for most.

AMA Guide to Prescription and OTC Drugs
Random House, 1988, 576 pages
One of the few full size hardcover references, this is a well-illustrated comprehensive reference that includes general information on diseases and how drugs work and pictures of many tablets and capsules. Good, usable information. Special notes on elderly use. Newer edition, if available, a must. 1988 edition leaves out too many drugs.

Consumer Guide to Prescription Drugs
Signet Reference, 1995, 1024 pages
Good value. Listed primarily by generic name, but with brand name cross-referencing. No consistent information on elderly.

The PDR Guide to Prescription Drugs
Medical Economics Data, 1994, 958 pages
Larger page size than most. Alphabetical by brand name only (index also available). Slightly different format than most others. Lacks OTC information. Some elderly information available. Expensive for the information available.

The Peoples Pharmacy
Joe Graedon
St. Martin's Paperbacks, 1985
Interesting information in unique presentation, but not useful as a comprehensive reference, and 1985 edition is outdated.

The Pill Book
Harold Silverman, Editor
Bantam Trade Paperback, 1994
Good general information, includes pictures of many pills. Elderly information included.

The Pill Guide
Lynn Sonberg
Berkeley Books, 1992
A good value, but this book lacks special information about use in elderly and information on newer drugs. Review ease of use before purchase.

USP Drug Information for the Consumer
Consumer Reports, with permission of USP (United States Pharmacopeia), 1990, 1761 pages
Large pages. An authoritative, comprehensive book, with pictures of many pills as well as more comprehensive identification codes for other drugs. Alphabetized by generic name only, with brand names listed in the index. 1990 edition means many new drugs not included.

Other References that Include Drug Information

Like this book, there are a number of references which include some information on drugs. Even when provided to the extent found in our *Medication Quick Reference,* medication information included in multipurpose books should be supplemented with more detailed references, even if they are not as easy to use. Do not forget the resources available to you through a full service pharmacy, but, if possible, you should do some research on your own before contacting the pharmacy.

More Technical References

As noted previously, there are many more drug references, including some for consumers. If you are a health care professional or employ a nurse, physician, or pharmacist to provide on-site services, one of the more technical references might be suitable. Ask the person who is employed or who visits his or her preferences. The publications listed below vary in price from around $25.00 to well over $100.00.

* *Nursing 96* (There is a new edition each year, with the last two digits of the year as part of the title.), widely used by nurses and published by *Nursing.* This is a soft-cover pocket sized reference that focuses on proper administration and observation for adverse effects.

- *Facts and Comparisons,* in a hard-cover or subscription loose leaf format, is a comprehensive reference of virtually all prescription and OTC drugs and widely used by pharmacists.

- *AMA Drug Evaluations,* published by the American Medical Association and available in soft cover (full-sized pages).

- *The Physicians Drug Reference* by Medical Economics Data, a difficult, but widely used reference because it is based solely on official manufacturer monographs for prescription drugs only (OTC and ophthalmic product versions that also simply use official product labeling are available as well).

- *American Hospital Formulary Service,* from the American Society of Hospital Pharmacists, in loose-leaf subscription format or hard-cover, similar in content and use to *Drug Facts and Comparisons.*

- *USP Drug Information,* from the USPC, is available in soft-cover (full sized) and includes comprehensive, authoritative information in multiple volumes.

- *American Pharmaceutical Association Geriatric Dosage Handbook,* Lexi-Comp Inc, is a useful publication of all geriatric health providers. It comes in a soft-cover handbook style and is conveniently formatted so that one can look up either generic or brand names alphabetically without using an index. Strong on geriatric considerations, much can be used by laypersons as well.

APPENDIX 5
Sample Residential Care Forms

Admission Agreement side one

ADMISSION AGREEMENT

In consideration of _____being admitted to the facility it is agreed as follows:
Rooms are rented on a 30 day basis. The resident admitted and /or guarantor agrees to pay on a month to month in advance basis the sum of \$_____per month, due and payable promptly on the lst of each month, commencing on _____ for board and care. There will be a l0% charge if payment is received after the 5th of the month. There is an annual 5-7% adjustment of the monthly rate.

PAYMENTS: Source of funding : Private____ SSI____

If the resident and/or the guarantor fails or refuses to pay, and it is necessary to place the account in the hands of a collection agency and/or attorney for collection, the resident or his guarantor agrees to pay all collection agency charges and expenses incurred by the court.

TRANSFER AND DISCHARGE

The resident shall not be transferred from the home without first giving 30 days written notice to the facility and paying all accrued charges.
In case the resident has to be admitted to a hospital or convalescent home, or expires, no refunds need by given, unless the room is rented to another resident, in which case the daily pro-rated rate will be refunded.
The home will give a 30 day written notice to the resident or guarantor if it becomes necessary to transfer a resident. However, in case of emergency conditions where the home feels residents health, safety, or the operations of the home are involved a three (3) day notice with the approval of CCL will given.
In case of annual and extra care cost increases, a 30 day written notice will be given to the resident or guarantor. At that time a new admission agreement will be signed by both parties.
We reserve the right to reassign rooms, should it become necessary.

Pro-rated to the lst of the month \$_____

SMOKING IN DESIGNATED AREAS ONLY.

PHYSICIAN REQUIRED

The personal physician of the resident is Dr._____, who may be called in attendance by the home at its discretion and if said doctor is not available, the home may call another doctor for the resident, any expense to be borne by the resident and/or guarantor.

RESTRICTIONS AND LIABILITIES

No food, liquids, or medicines shall be brought into the home for the resident without permission first having been obtained from the home. All personal property both incoming and outgoing shall be recorded on the inventory sheet and signed by all parties.

Admission Agreement side two

.1) BASIC GENERAL SERVICES:
    A) Lodging: Single room_____ Double room_____
    B) Food Services:
       a. Three nutritious meals daily, and between meal nourishment or snacks.
       b. Special diets if prescribed by a doctor.
2) BASIC PERSONAL SERVICES:
       a. Laundry service and cleaning of the residents room.
       b. Comfortable and suitable bed, including fresh linen weekly or more often if
          needed.
       c. Plan, arrange and / or provide for transportation to medical and dental
          appointments.
       d. Notification to family and other appropriate person / agency of clients needs.
       e. Continuous observation, care, and supervision, as required.
       f. Assistance in meeting necessary medical and dental needs.
       g. Assistance, as needed, with taking prescribed medications in accordance
          with physicians instructions, unless prohibited by law or regulation.
       h. A planned activity program, including arrangement for utilization of available
          community resources.
       i. Assistance with bathing and personal needs, as required.
       j. Bedside care for minor temporary illnesses.
       k. The facility will not handle residents funds or act as sub-payee.

OPTIONAL SERVICES
       a. Incontinent care bladder $ per mo. in advance; does not include supplies.
       b. Incontinent care bladder and bowel $ per mo. in advance does not include supplies.
       c. Regular tray service $ per meal in advance.
       d. Standby assistance with transferring and ambulation $ per mo. in advance.

3) VISITING HOURS
       a. Hours are between 10:00am and 8:00pm.
       b. Family and friends are encouraged to have meals with residents with advance notice.

State Licensing Agency, CCL, has the right to interview and review residents records at any time.
The undersigned has read, understands, and agrees to the terms and conditions of this contract.

DATED:_____ RESIDENT:_____

GUARANTOR:_____

ADDRESS:_____

PHONE:(H) (____)_____ (W) (____)_____

TOTAL MONTHLY CHARGE $_____ ADMITTED BY_____

Copies received by resident or responsible person of admission agreement, personal rights,personal
property policy and house rules.

Signature_____Date_____

STATE OF CALIFORNIA — HEALTH AND WELFARE AGENCY

DEPARTMENT OF SOCIAL SERVICES
COMMUNITY CARE LICENSING

CLIENT/RESIDENT PERSONAL PROPERTY AND VALUABLES

Facilities must safeguard client's/resident's personal property/valuables entrusted to the facility. Licensee/Administrator is responsible for maintaining a record of personal property/valuables entrusted to and removed from the facility. Under "Number", enter the quantity of items entrusted. Under "Description", describe the item (marking articles by names or numbers may aid identification.). Under "Location", enter where items are stored. Licensee/Administrator and client/resident must sign each entry. Explain why, if client/resident does not sign. Provide a copy to the client/resident and maintain a copy in client's/resident's file. As property/valuable is removed, explain the reason for removal, enter the removal date, and ensure form is signed by all required persons specified above.

The reverse side of this form may be completed and retained in Residential Care Facilities for the Elderly to meet the notice requirements of Health and Safety Code Section 1569.153(k).

Name of Client/Resident	Social Security No.

A. PERSONAL PROPERTY/VALUABLES ENTRUSTED TO FACILITY

Number	Description	Date	Location	Signature of Client/Resident (or if "None" explain) / Signature of Licensee/Administrator

B. PERSONAL PROPERTY/VALUABLES REMOVED

Number	Description	Date	Location	Signature of Client/Resident (or if "None" explain) / Signature of Licensee/Administrator

STATE OF CALIFORNIA
HEALTH AND WELFARE AGENCY

DEPARTMENT OF SOCIAL SERVICES
COMMUNITY CARE LICENSING

IDENTIFICATION AND EMERGENCY INFORMATION

This information is required under the H & S Code and the regulations of the Department to be maintained on every person admitted to a community care facility, to be readily available to the person in charge, but not accessible to unauthorized persons. All information must be kept current. See other side for additional information required for residential facilities for children.

A. ALL FACILITIES (EXCEPT CHILD CARE FACILITIES; COMPLETE LIC 700)

1. NAME OF CLIENT OR CHILD		SOCIAL SECURITY NUMBER (OPTIONAL)	DATE OF BIRTH	AGE	SEX
2. RESPONSIBLE PERSON OR PLACEMENT AGENCY		ADDRESS		TELEPHONE ( )	
3. NAME OF NEAREST RELATIVE (OPTIONAL)	RELATIONSHIP	ADDRESS		TELEPHONE ( )	
4. DATE ADMITTED TO FACILITY	ADDRESS PRIOR TO ADMISSION				
5. DATE LEFT	FORWARDING ADDRESS				
6. REASONS FOR LEAVING FACILITY					

7. **PERSON(S) RESPONSIBLE FOR FINANCIAL AFFAIRS, PAYMENT FOR CARE, LEGAL GUARDIAN, IF ANY**

NAME	ADDRESS	TELEPHONE
		( )
		( )
		( )

8. **OTHER PERSONS TO BE NOTIFIED IN EMERGENCY**

NAME	ADDRESS	TELEPHONE
a. PHYSICIAN		( )
b. MENTAL HEALTH PROVIDER, IF ANY		( )
c. DENTIST		( )
d. RELATIVE(S)		( )
e. FRIEND(S)		( )

9. **EMERGENCY HOSPITALIZATION PLAN**

NAME OF HOSPITAL TO BE TAKEN IN AN EMERGENCY	ADDRESS OF HOSPITAL TO BE TAKEN IN AN EMERGENCY
MEDICAL PLAN	MEDICAL PLAN IDENTIFICATION NUMBER
NAME OF DENTAL PLAN (IF ANY)	DENTAL PLAN NUMBER (IF ANY)

10. **OTHER REQUIRED INFORMATION**

a. AMBULATORY STATUS

b. RELIGIOUS PREFERENCE	NAME AND ADDRESS OF CLERGYMAN OR RELIGIOUS ADVISOR, IF ANY	TELEPHONE ( )

11. COMMENTS

Physician's Report side one

STATE OF CALIFORNIA – HEALTH AND WELFARE AGENCY

DEPARTMENT OF SOCIAL SERVICES
COMMUNITY CARE LICENSING

PHYSICIAN'S REPORT FOR COMMUNITY CARE FACILITIES
For Resident/Client Of, Or Applicants For Admission To, Community Care Facilities (CCF).

NOTE TO PHYSICIAN:
The person specified below is a resident/client of or an applicant for admission to a licensed Community Care Facility. These types of facilities are currently responsible for providing the level of care and supervision, primarily nonmedical care, necessary to meet the needs of the individual residents/clients.

THESE FACILITIES DO NOT PROVIDE PROFESSIONAL NURSING CARE.
The information that you complete on this person is required by law to assist in determining whether he/she is appropriate for admission to or continued care in a facility.

FACILITY INFORMATION (To be completed by the licensee/designee)

NAME OF FACILITY: TELEPHONE:

ADDRESS: NUMBER   STREET   CITY

LICENSEE'S NAME: TELEPHONE: FACILITY LICENSE NUMBER:

RESIDENT/CLIENT INFORMATION (To be completed by the resident/authorized representative/licensee)

NAME: TELEPHONE:

ADDRESS: NUMBER   STREET   CITY   SOCIAL SECURITY NUMBER:

NEXT OF KIN: PERSON RESPONSIBLE FOR THIS PERSON'S FINANCES:

PATIENT'S DIAGNOSIS (To be completed by the physician)

PRIMARY DIAGNOSIS:

SECONDARY DIAGNOSIS: LENGTH OF TIME UNDER YOUR CARE:

AGE:	HEIGHT:	SEX:	WEIGHT:	IN YOUR OPINION DOES THIS PERSON REQUIRE SKILLED NURSING CARE? ☐ YES ☐ NO

TUBERCULOSIS EXAMINATION RESULTS: ☐ ACTIVE   ☐ INACTIVE   ☐ NONE   DATE OF LAST TB TEST:

TYPE OF TB TEST USED: TREATMENT/MEDICATION: ☐ YES ☐ NO   If YES, list below:

OTHER CONTAGIOUS/INFECTIOUS DISEASES:
A)   ☐ YES   ☐ NO   If YES, list below:

TREATMENT/MEDICATION:
B)   ☐ YES   ☐ NO   If YES, list below:

ALLERGIES
C)   ☐ YES   ☐ NO   If YES, list below:

TREATMENT/MEDICATION:
D)   ☐ YES   ☐ NO   If YES, list below:

Ambulatory status of client/resident: ☐ Ambulatory   ☐ Nonambulatory

Health and Safety Code Section 13131 provides: "Nonambulatory persons" means persons unable to leave a building unassisted under emergency conditions. It includes any person who is unable, or likely to be unable, to physically and mentally respond to a sensory signal approved by the State Fire Marshal, or an oral instruction relating to fire danger, and persons who depend upon mechanical aids such as crutches, walkers, and wheelchairs. The determination of ambulatory or nonambulatory status of persons with developmental disabilities shall be made by the Director of Social Services or his or her designated representative, in consultation with the Director of Developmental Services or his or her designated representative. The determination of ambulatory or nonambulatory status of all other disabled persons placed after January 1, 1984, who are not developmentally disabled shall be made by the Director of Social Services, or his or her designated representative.

LIC 602 (3/94)   *(OVER)*   94 26822

Physician's Report side two

I. PHYSICAL HEALTH STATUS: ☐ GOOD ☐ FAIR ☐ POOR	COMMENTS:			
	YES NO (Check One)	ASSISTIVE DEVICE		COMMENTS:
1. Auditory Impairment				
2. Visual Impairment				
3. Wears Dentures				
4. Special Diet				
5. Substance Abuse Problem				
6. Bowel Impairment				
7. Bladder Impairment				
8. Motor Impairment				
9. Requires Continuous Bed Care				

II. MENTAL HEALTH STATUS: ☐ GOOD ☐ FAIR ☐ POOR	COMMENTS:			
	NO PROBLEM	OCCASIONAL	FREQUENT	IF PROBLEM EXISTS, PROVIDE COMMENT BELOW:
1. Confused				
2. Able To Follow Instructions				
3. Depressed				
4. Able to Communicate				

III. CAPACITY FOR SELF CARE: ☐ YES ☐ NO	COMMENTS:	
	YES NO (Check One)	COMMENTS:
1. Able to care For All Personal Needs		
2. Can Administer and Store Own Medications		
3. Needs Constant Medical Supervision		
4. Currently Taking Prescribed Medications		
5. Bathes Self		
6. Dresses Self		
7. Feeds Self		
8. Cares For His/Her Own Toilet Needs		
9. Able to Leave Facility Unassisted		
10. Able to Ambulate Without Assistance		

PLEASE LIST OVER-THE-COUNTER MEDICATION THAT CAN BE GIVEN TO THE CLIENT/RESIDENT, AS NEEDED, FOR THE FOLLOWING CONDITIONS:

CONDITIONS   **OVER-THE-COUNTER MEDICATION(S)**

1. Headache
2. Constipation
3. Diarrhea
4. Indigestion
5. Others *(specify condition)*

PLEASE LIST CURRENT <u>PRESCRIBED MEDICATIONS</u> THAT ARE BEING TAKEN BY CLIENT/RESIDENT:

1. _____   4. _____   7. _____
2, _____   5. _____   8. _____
3. _____   6. _____   9. _____

PHYSICIAN'S NAME AND ADDRESS:	TELEPHONE:	DATE:

PHYSICIAN'S SIGNATURE

AUTHORIZATION FOR RELEASE OF MEDICAL INFORMATION (TO BE COMPLETED BY PERSON'S AUTHORIZED REPRESENTATIVE)
I hereby authorize the release of medical information contained in this report regarding the physical examination of:

PATIENT'S NAME:

TO (NAME AND ADDRESS OF LICENSING AGENCY):

SIGNATURE OF RESIDENT/POTENTIAL RESIDENT AND/OR HIS/HER AUTHORIZED REPRESENTATIVE	ADDRESS:	DATE:

Unusual Incident/Injury/Death Report side one

STATE OF CALIFORNIA - HEALTH AND WELFARE AGENCY

DEPARTMENT OF SOCIAL SERVICES
COMMUNITY CARE LICENSING

UNUSUAL INCIDENT/INJURY/ DEATH REPORT

INSTRUCTIONS TO THE FACILITY LICENSEE: NOTIFY THE LICENSING AGENCY WITHIN THE AGENCY'S NEXT WORKING DAY AND, AS APPLICABLE, PERSON(S) AND/OR PLACEMENT AGENCY(IES) RESPONSIBLE FOR CLIENT(S)/RESIDENT(S) OF ANY UNUSUAL EVENT, INCIDENT, INJURY OR DEATH REQUIRING MEDICAL TREATMENT AS DETERMINED BY THE PHYSICIAN. COMPLETE AND RETURN THE ORIGINAL COPY OF THIS FORM TO THE LICENSING AGENCY WITHIN SEVEN (7) DAYS OF THE EVENT. RETAIN A COPY IN THE CLIENT'S/RESIDENT'S FILE. IF ADDITIONAL SPACE IS NEEDED, PLEASE ATTACH SHEET(S).
NOTE: RESIDENTIAL CARE FACILITIES FOR THE ELDERLY SHALL COMPLY WITH CALIFORNIA CODE OF REGULATIONS, SECTION 87561 PERTAINING TO THESE REPORTING REQUIREMENTS.

NAME OF FACILITY

FACILITY FILE NUMBER

TELEPHONE NUMBER
(   )

ADDRESS

CLIENTS/RESIDENTS INVOLVED	DATE OCCURRED	CHECK APPROPRIATE BOX			AGE	SEX	DATE OF ADMISSION
		UNUSUAL INCIDENT	INJURY	DEATH			
1.							
2.							
3.							
4.							

I. **UNUSUAL EVENT OR INCIDENT** - UNUSUAL INCIDENTS INCLUDE CLIENT/RESIDENT ABUSE, UNEXPLAINED ABSENCES, OR ANYTHING THAT AFFECTS THE PHYSICAL OR EMOTIONAL HEALTH OR SAFETY OF ANY CLIENT/RESIDENT AND EPIDEMIC OUTBREAKS, POISONINGS, CATASTROPHES, FACILITY FIRES OR EXPLOSIONS.

DESCRIBE EVENT OR INCIDENT *(INCLUDE DATE, TIME, LOCATION, NATURE OF INCIDENT, AND HOW CLIENTS/RESIDENTS WERE AFFECTED)*

EXPLAIN WHAT IMMEDIATE ACTION WAS TAKEN *(INCLUDE PERSONS CONTACTED AND IF INJURY OCCURRED COMPLETE SECTION II)*

DESCRIBE WHAT FOLLOW-UP ACTION IS PLANNED *(INCLUDE STEPS TAKEN TO PREVENT REOCCURRENCE)*

II. **INJURY REQUIRING MEDICAL TREATMENT**

DESCRIBE HOW, WHERE AND TO WHOM INJURY OCCURRED

LIC 624 (11/89) (CONFIDENTIAL)

89 55329

Unusual Incident/Injury/Death Report side two

WHAT APPEARS TO BE THE EXTENT OF THE INJURIES TO CLIENT/RESIDENTS?

PERSON(S) WHO OBSERVED THE INJURY

ATTENDING PHYSICIAN'S NAME, FINDINGS, AND TREATMENT

III. DEATH REPORT

DATE AND TIME OF DEATH	DECEASED CLIENT/RESIDENT	PLACE OF DEATH

DESCRIBE IMMEDIATE CAUSE OF DEATH *(IF CORONER REPORT MADE, SEND COPY WITHIN 30 DAYS)*

DESCRIBE CONDITIONS CONTRIBUTING TO DEATH

WHAT ACTION DID YOU TAKE?

NAME OF ATTENDING PHYSICIAN

NAME OF MORTICIAN

SIGNATURE OF PERSON REPORTING	DATE
▶	
SIGNATURE OF LICENSEE/ADMINISTRATOR	DATE
▶	

Glossary

Activities of Daily Living   Abilities and skills needed for independent living, such as ability to bathe, use the toilet, prepare and eat meals, and dress.

Acute Disease   Having a sudden onset; sharp or severe.

Angina   Usually used in reference to angina pectoris, a type of chest pain associated with coronary artery disease; most commonly a crushing pain located in the center of the chest, but also may be associated with pain in the shoulder, back, jaw, or arm and may be accompanied by or experienced only as a sensation of numbness in these areas.

Ambulation   Walking or moving about.

Aspiration   Inhaling a foreign material, such as food, medication, or vomit into the lungs; large matter may cause choking, while smaller matter may cause coughing, and if the material is not evacuated from the airways it may lead to lung infection.

Assistive Devices   Usually used in reference to ambulation devices, such as cane, walker, or crutches, but also used in reference to such safety devices as handrails, grab bars, or over-the-bed trapeze.

Bacteria   One-celled, microscopic organisms, some of which are responsible for human disease.

Blood Clot   Accumulation of blood products and components; when located within the interior of a blood vessel, a blood clot is referred to as a thrombus.

Bronchi   Plural for bronchus; refers to the two main branches of airway leading into the lung from the trachea.

Bronchitis   Inflammation of the lining of one or both bronchi.

Chronic Illness   A disease that lasts for a long time, often for the rest of a person's life, as in diabetes, high blood pressure, and kidney failure.

Coma   A deep state of unconsciousness in which the individual exhibits no response to painful stimuli and is lacking in normal reflexive movements.

Contracture   Abnormal shortening of muscle tissues, making stretching and normal full extension of muscle difficult to impossible.

Dementia   Decrease in intellectual function, resulting in losses in memory, learning, and recall ability.

Depression   A mental state characterized by feelings of extreme sadness and hopelessness.

Diabetes   A disease in which the ability of the body to control the level of sugar in the blood is impaired; sometimes referred to as sugar diabetes, but its proper name is diabetes mellitus.

Dialysis   A procedure used to filter waste products from the blood when the kidneys are no longer able to accomplish this function; may be performed extracorporeally (outside the body) using a dialysis machine connected to the body's circulation, or intracorporeally (inside the body) using the peritoneal membrane which lines the abdomen.

Distention   Bloating as with fluid or air; may be used to refer to bladder distention when the bladder is unable to empty urine or to abdominal distention when abdominal organs are distended with fluid, an enlarged organ or other structure, or solid waste.

Drug Interaction   The effect of one drug on another in the body; may result in a reduced or increased effect of one or both drugs, or may produce severe reactions that in themselves require medical attention.

Drug-Diet Interactions	The effect of a drug on appetite, which may be increased or decreased as a result.
Drug-Food Interactions	The effect of food on the absorption, utilization, or clearance of a drug from the body.
Enema	The introduction of water, either tap or salty, into the rectum to soften the stool and stimulate a bowel movement; some enemas are prepared with drugs to either stimulate the bowel or draw extra water into the bowel.
Filtration	Process of removing undesired elements from a mixture, as in kidney filtration in which excess chemical elements and waste products are removed from the blood.
Fungus	A vegetative cellular growth, including yeasts and molds.
Gout	An acute form of arthritis, usually affecting the great toe, heel, and ankle, causing redness, swelling, tenderness, and formation of sharp microscopic crystals in the joint fluid.
Incontinence	Undesired, involuntary loss of urine or stool of sufficient frequency or severity to be a problem.
Inflammation	The body's reaction to injury; may be caused by chemical, bacterial, viral, mechanical, or toxic processes.
Insulin	A hormone produced in the pancreas that helps maintain normal blood sugar levels.
Mental Illness	A disease that affects the brain, which controls thinking ability, mood, appetite, and sleeping.
Mental Status	Quality of thought and feeling in relation to circumstances.
Migraine	A sensitivity of the blood vessels around the brain that results in severe headaches, often preceded or accompanied by a sensory disturbance called an aura.

Ombudsman	Individual who serves as state liason and advocate for persons living in a nursing home.
Ostomy	A new opening in the skin created surgically to drain the natural body excretions of urine or stool.
Physical Therapy	Treatment directed at restoration of normal musculoskeletal alignment and function.
Pneumonia	An infection of the lungs.
Pox	A type of rash characterized by fluid- or pus-filled skin eruptions.
PRN	"As needed;" in reference to scheduling doses of a medication.
Prosthesis	Artificial limb or body part such as artificial hip.
Range of Motion	Degree of movement in each direction that is possible for head, trunk, and extremities in normal postures.
Rehabilitation	Treatment measures taken to restore functions that have been impaired by illness or injury.
Routine Medication	Medication taken on a daily or other regular basis to maintain control over disease process; also referred to as maintenance medication.
Scar Tissue	Replacement tissue that forms over injured skin or body organ following changes caused by injury, disease, or surgery.
Sepsis	Presence of microscopic organisms or their by-products in the bloodstream; can represent a life-threatening infectious process.
Shunt	An artificial connection designed to allow access to or relief of a bodily structure; an arteriovenous shunt is used to gain access to the circulation for dialysis; a cranial shunt is used to relieve fluid pressure on the brain.
Side-effects	Actions of a drug that are not part of the desired, or therapeutic, effect.

Sleep Apnea   Interruption of normal breathing during sleep.

Speech Therapy   Program of treatment designed to improve ability to speak and vocalize, for example, following a stroke; treatment program planned and implemented by a speech therapist.

Stable Angina   Angina pectoris that is predictable in onset, severity, duration, and method of relief; usually managed with medication.

Therapeutic Effects Desired, or intended, effects of a medication.

Unstable Angina   Angina pectoris that is not predictable or changes from a predictable pattern by becoming more severe, spreading to other parts of the body, occurring more often or as a result of lesser factors.

Variant Angina   Angina pectoris that is not characterized by chest pain and may cause nausea, shortness of breath, or dizziness.

Virus   Microscopic organism, similar to bacteria in that it is capable of producing disease in humans.

Vital Signs   Measurements of vital organ function; blood pressure, pulse, temperature, and respiratory rate.

A

Abdominal pain, 44-50
Acceptance of residents, 26-29
Accidental falls, 112-115
Accupril, guidelines for, 234
ACE inhibitors; *see* Angiotensin converting enzyme inhibitors
Acetaminophen
  for arthritis, 61
  for broken bones, 74
  for cancer, 79
  for fever and chills, 117, 119
  guidelines for, 234
  for headache, 121, 122
  for muscle or bone pain, 143, 144
Acetaminophen with codeine, guidelines for, 234
Acetazolamide, guidelines for, 234
Acetophenazine, guidelines for, 234
Acetylsalicylic acid, guidelines for, 238
Achromycin, guidelines for, 234
Acid-blocking agents, for abdominal pain, 47
Activities of daily living
  difficulties with, 8
  sample care plan and, 33, 35
Activity level
  angina and, 55
  ankle swelling and, 61
  arthritis and, 64
  cancer and, 82
  congestive heart failure and, 86
  dementia and, 101
  diabetes and, 107
  fever and chills and, 119
  heart attack and, 126, 128

  high blood pressure and, 132
  movement disorders and, 141
  seizures and, 141
  shortness of breath and, 177
  stroke and, 182
Acular, guidelines for, 234
Acyclovir, for rash, 167
Adalat, guidelines for, 235
Adapin, guidelines for, 235
Adhesions, 49-50
ADLs; *see* Activities of daily living
Administration of medications, 208-225
  buccal, 212
  in ears, 217-219
  in eyes, 214-217
  nasal, 219-222
  oral, 208-212
  rectal, 222-224
  sublingual, 212
  topical, 224-225
  transdermal, 212-214
  vaginal, 224
Admission records, 27
Adrenalin, guidelines for, 235
Adult day health care centers, 20-21
Adverse drug reactions, 195, 228
Advil; *see* Ibuprofen
Advocacy programs, 19
AeroBid, guidelines for, 235; *see also* Flunisolide
Afrin, guidelines for, 235
Air mattresses, for pressure ulcers, 156
Akineton, guidelines for, 235
Albuterol
  for cough, 94
  guidelines for, 235

  in inhalers, 221
  for shortness of breath, 175
Alcohol
  headache from, 123
  sleep problems and, 153
Alcoholic dementia, 97
Aldactazide, guidelines for, 235
Aldactone, guidelines for, 235
Aldomet, guidelines for, 235; *see also* Methylda
Alginates, for pressure ulcers, 155, 157
Alginic acid, guidelines for, 235
Allergic drug reactions, 195
Allopurinol
  for arthritis, 62
  guidelines for, 235
Alpha blockers, for high blood pressure, 131
Alprazolam
  guidelines for, 235
  for psychiatric disorders, 162
Altace, guidelines for, 235
Aluminum antacids, for kidney failure, 135
Aluminum carbonate, guidelines for, 236
Aluminum hydroxide
  for abdominal pain, 47
  guidelines for, 236
Alupent, guidelines for, 236
Alzheimer's disease, dementia and, 97
Amantadine, guidelines for, 236
Ambenyl, guidelines for, 236
Ambien, guidelines for, 236; *see also* Zolpidem
American Cancer Society's Warning Signs of Cancer, 78
American Hospital Association, on patient's bill of rights, 16-17

Amitriptyline, guidelines for, 236
Amoxapine, guidelines for, 236
Amoxicillin, guidelines for, 236
Amoxicillin-clavulanate, guide lines for, 236
Amphogel; *see* Aluminum antacids
Ampicillin
    guidelines for, 236
    for urinary incontinence, 68
Anacin; *see* Acetaminophen
Analgesics
    for abdominal pain, 47
    for ankle swelling, 57
    for arthritis, 61-62
    for broken bones, 74
    for cancer, 79
    for fever and chills, 117
    for headache, 121
    for muscle or bone pain, 143
    over-the-counter, 232
Anaprox, guidelines for, 236
Ancobon, guidelines for, 236
Anexsia, guidelines for, 236
Angina, 51-55
Angiotensin converting enzyme inhibitors
    for angina, 53
    for ankle swelling, 57
    for congestive heart failure, 84
    cough from, 93
    guidelines for, 234
    for heart attack, 125-126
    for high blood pressure, 130
Ankle swelling, 56-59
    in congestive heart failure, 85-86
Ansaid, guidelines for, 237
Anspor, guidelines for, 237
Antacids
    for abdominal pain, 47
    diarrhea from, 108

guidelines for, 236
    for kidney failure, 135
    over-the-counter, 231-232
Antianxiety drugs
    for dementia, 99
    for psychiatric disorders, 162
Antibiotics
    for cough, 94, 96
    for diarrhea, 96
    diarrhea from, 108
    in eye medications, 215
    purpose of, 192
    for rash, 167
    topical, over-the-counter, 233
    for ulcers, 49
    for urinary incontinence, 68
Anticholinergics
    guidelines for, 237
    for urinary incontinence, 67
Anticonvulsants, for seizures, 139
Antidepressants
    hot weather and, 118
    for psychiatric disorders, 161, 163
    tricyclic, 273
Antidiarrheal drugs, 109
Antiemetics, for nausea and vomiting, 147
Antiepileptics, for stroke, 180
Antifungal drugs
    for rash, 167
    topical, over-the-counter, 233
Antihistamines
    guidelines for, 237
    hot weather and, 118
Antinausea drugs, for cancer, 79
Antiparkinson drugs
    hot weather and, 118

for movement disorders, 139
Antipsychotics
    for dementia, 99
    guidelines for, 237
    hot weather and, 118
    for psychiatric disorders, 162
Antipyretics, for fever and chills, 117
Antirejection drugs, for kidney failure, 135
Antiseptics, topical, over-the-counter, 233
Antispasmotics, for abdominal pain, 47
Antituberculosis drugs, for cough, 94
Antivert, guidelines for, 238
Antiviral drugs, for rash, 167
Anxiety
    in dementia, 89, 99
    as psychiatric disorder, 160, 161
    sleep problems and, 150
APAP, guidelines for, 238
Appetite, effect of drugs on, 197-198
Apresoline, guidelines for, 238
Artane, guidelines for, 238
Arthritis, 60-64
Artificial tears, 215
    guidelines for, 238
"As Needed" medications, 193-195
    sample administration form for, 196
    scheduling of, 202
ASA, guidelines for, 234
Asendin, guidelines for, 238
Aspiration, in nausea and vomiting, 146
Aspirin
    for arthritis, 61

for broken bones, 74
for cancer, 79
for fever and chills, 117, 119
guidelines for, 238
for headache, 121, 122
for muscle or bone pain,
 142, 143, 144
for stroke, 180
Assistance, types of, 11
Associations, as resource for
 help, 22-23
Astemizole, guidelines for, 238
Atarax, guidelines for, 238
Atenolol
 for angina, 53
 guidelines for, 238
 for heart attack, 126
 for high blood pressure, 130
Atherosclerosis, 51-55
Ativan, guidelines for, 238;
 see also Lorazepam
Atrial fibrillation, stroke and,
 178
Atropine
 for abdominal pain, 47
 guidelines for, 238
Atrovent, guidelines for, 239;
 see also Ipratropium
Attapulgite, guidelines for, 238
Attitude of staff, 12
Audit process, 228-229
Augmentin, guidelines for, 239
Aventyl, guidelines for, 239
Axis, guidelines for, 239
Azithromycin, guidelines for,
 239
Azmacort; *see also*
 Triamcinolone
 guidelines for, 239
 for shortness of breath, 175

B
Bacampicillin, guidelines for,
 239

Baclofen, guidelines for, 239
Bactrim, guidelines for, 239;
 see also Trimethoprim/
 sulfamethoxazole
Bactroban, guidelines for, 239
Balance disorders, 170-173
Basaljel, guidelines for, 239
Bayer; *see* Aspirin
Beclomethasone
 for cough, 94
 guidelines for, 239
 in inhalers, 221-222
Beclovent; *see* Beclomethasone
 Beepen VK, guidelines
 for, 239
Behavior problems, in demen-
 tia, 101
Belladonna
 for abdominal pain, 47
 guidelines for, 239
Benadryl, guidelines for, 239
Benazepril, guidelines for, 239
Benemid, guidelines for, 240;
 see also Probenecid
Bentyl, guidelines for, 240
Benzocaine, guidelines for,
 240
Benzodiazepines, guidelines
 for, 240
Benzonatate, for cough, 94
Benztropine, guidelines for,
 240
Bepridil, guidelines for, 240
Beta blockers
 for angina, 53
 guidelines for, 240
 for headache, 122
 for heart attack, 125, 126
 for high blood pressure, 130
Betagan, guidelines for, 240
Bethanechol
 guidelines for, 241
 for urinary incontinence, 67

Biaxin, guidelines for, 241
Biperiden, guidelines for, 241
Bisacodyl, guidelines for, 241
Bismuth subsalicylate, guide-
 lines for, 241
Bladder problems, 65-71
Bleeding, from constipation,
 87
Bleph-10, guidelines for, 241
Blindness, 170
Blocadren, guidelines for, 241
Blood, vomiting of, 147
Blood pressure, high, 129-132
Blood sugar, diabetes and,
 102-107
Blood tests, adverse drug reac-
 tions and, 195
Body temperature, fever and
 chills and, 116-119
Body weight
 arthritis and, 64
 kidney failure and, 134
Bone pain, 142-145
Bones, broken, 72-76
Bowel pain; *see* Abdominal pain
Bowels; *see* Stools
Brain, stroke and, 178, 182
Brain diseases, movement dis-
 orders and seizures and, 137
Breath, shortness of, 175-177
Broken bones, 72-76
Bromocriptine
 guidelines for, 241
 for movement disorders, 139
Bromodiphenhydramine,
 guidelines for, 241
Brompheniramine, guidelines
 for, 241
Bronchitis, cough and, 93
Bronchodilators
 for cough, 94
 guidelines for, 241
 for shortness of breath, 175

Bruises, in muscle or bone
    pain, 145
Buccal medications, 212, 213
Bumex, guidelines for, 242
Bupropion, guidelines for, 242
BuSpar, guidelines for, 242;
    see also Buspirone
Buspirone
    for dementia, 99
    for psychiatric disorders, 162

C

Cafergot; *see* Ergot
Caffeine
    for headache, 122
    withdrawal headache and,
        121, 123
Calan, guidelines for, 242;
    see also Verapamil
Calcium, drug interactions
    with, 197
Calcium carbonate
    for abdominal pain, 47
    guidelines for, 242
Calcium channel blockers
    for angina, 53
    guidelines for, 242
    for heart attack, 125, 126
    for high blood pressure, 130
Cancer, 77-82
Capoten, guidelines for, 242;
    see also Captopril
Capsaicin, guidelines for, 242
Capsules, 208
Captopril, for high blood
    pressure, 130
Carafate, guidelines for, 243;
    see also Sucralfate
Carbachol, guidelines for, 243
Carbamazepine
    guidelines for, 243
    for seizures, 139
Carbanide peroxide, for ear
    disorders, 171

Carbenicillin, guidelines for,
    243
Carbidopa
    guidelines for, 256
    for sleep problems, 151
Cardene, guidelines for, 243
Cardizem, guidelines for, 243;
    see also Diltiazem
Cardura; *see* Doxazosin
Care plans, 30-32
    sample, 33-36
Caregivers; *see also* Staff
    checklist for abilities of, 15
    finding good ones, 13-14
    orientation and training of,
        14-15
    where to look for, 13
Carteolol, guidelines for, 243
Casanthranol, guidelines for,
    243
Casts for broken bones, 72,
    75, 76
Catapres; *see also* Clonidine
    guidelines for, 243
    in skin patch, 214
Cataracts, 172
Catheterization, urinary,
    incontinence and, 71
Ceclor, guidelines for, 243
Cefadroxil, guidelines for, 243
Cefixime, guidelines for, 244
Cefpodoxime, guidelines for,
    244
Cefprozil, guidelines for, 244
Ceftin, guidelines for, 244
Cephalexin
    guidelines for, 244
    for rash, 167
Cephradine, guidelines for,
    244
Cephulac, guidelines for, 244
Certified nursing assistants, 13
Chemical restraint, for
    dementia, 99

Chemotherapy, 79
Chest pain, 51-55
    in heart attack, 125, 128
Child resistant packaging, 200
Chills, 116-119
Chlor-trimeton, guidelines for,
    244
Chloral hydrate, guidelines
    for, 244
Chloramphenicol, guidelines
    for, 244
Chlordiazepoxide, guidelines
    for, 244
Chloroptic, guidelines for, 244
Chlorpheniramine, guidelines
    for, 244
Chlorpromazine, guidelines
    for, 244
Chlorthalidone, guidelines
    for, 244
Chlorzoxazone, guidelines for,
    245
Choledyl, guidelines for, 245
Cholestyramine, guidelines
    for, 245
Choline magnesium salicylate,
    guidelines for, 245
Cholinergics, for urinary
    incontinence, 67
Chronulac, guidelines for, 245
Churches, as resource for help,
    21-22
Ciloxan, guidelines for, 245
Cimetidine
    for abdominal pain, 47
    guidelines for, 245
Cipro, guidelines for, 245;
    see also Ciprofloxacin
Ciprofloxacin
    guidelines for, 245
    for urinary incontinence, 68
Civic groups, as resource for
    help, 22

Clarithromycin, guidelines for, 245

Clemastine, guidelines for, 245

Cleocin, guidelines for, 245

Clindamycin, guidelines for, 245

Clonazepam, guidelines for, 246

Clonidine
  guidelines for, 246
  for high blood pressure, 131

Clorazepate, guidelines for, 246

Closed fracture, 73

Clotrimazole, guidelines for, 246

Cloxacillin, guidelines for, 246

Clozapine, guidelines for, 246

CNAs; *see* Certified nursing assistants

Codeine
  for arthritis, 62
  for cancer, 79
  for cough, 94
  for headache, 121
  for muscle or bone pain, 143

Cogentin, guidelines for, 246

Cognex, guidelines for, 246;
  see also Tacrine

Colace, guidelines for, 246

Colchicine, for arthritis, 62

Cold application, for muscle or bone pain, 144

Cold medications, over-the-counter, 232

Colestid, guidelines for, 246

Community services/agencies, as resource for help, 20

Compazine, guidelines for, 246; *see also* Prochlorperazine

Compliance with medication, 227-228

Compoz; *see* Diphenhydramine

Compression fractures of spine, 142

Conduct, rules of, 12-13

Confusion, dementia and, 97-101

Congestive heart failure, 83-86
  ankle swelling and, 57
  cough and, 93
  shortness of breath and, 174

Conjugated estrogen
  guidelines for, 246
  for urinary incontinence, 67

Constipation, 87-91
  diarrhea from, 108, 111

Corgard, guidelines for, 246

Coronary arteries, heart attack and, 124

Coronary artery disease, 51-55

Cortisone, in eye medications, 215

Costs
  of medications, 227
  of residential care facilities, 5

Cough, 92-96

Cough medications
  over-the-counter, 232
  suppressants, 94

Coumadin, guidelines for, 246

Cozaar; *see* Losartan

Cromolyn, in inhalers, 222

Crushing tablets, 210-212

Cyclobenzaprine, guidelines for, 246

Cyclosporine, for kidney failure, 135

Cyproheptadine, guidelines for, 247

Cytotec, guidelines for, 247

Cytovene, guidelines for, 247

D

Dalmane, guidelines for, 247

Dantrolene, guidelines for, 247

Darvocet-N, guidelines for, 247

Daypro, guidelines for, 247

Debrox; *see*[Carbanide peroxide

Decadron, guidelines for, 247

Declomycin, guidelines for, 247

Degenerative arthritis, 60

Dehydration
  from diarrhea, 108
  in nausea and vomiting, 146

Delayed-release medications, 210

Demecarium, guidelines for, 247

Demeclocycline, guidelines for, 247

Dementia, 97-101
  incidence of, 7

Demerol, guidelines for, 247

Depakene, guidelines for, 247

Depakote, guidelines for, 248

Depression, 160-164

Desipramine
  guidelines for, 248
  for psychiatric disorders, 161

Desyrel, guidelines for, 248

Dexamethasone, guidelines for, 248

Dextromethorphan
  for cough, 94
  guidelines for, 248

D.H.E. 45; *see* Ergot

DiaBeta, guidelines for, 248

Diabetes, 102-107
  weakness or numbness and, 183, 184

Diabetic coma, 102
Dialysis, for kidney failure, 133-134
Diamox; *see* Acetazolamide
Diarrhea, 108-111
  from constipation, 87-88
Diazepam
  guidelines for, 248
  for psychiatric disorders, 162
Diclofenac, guidelines for, 248
Dicloxacillin, guidelines for, 248
Dicyclomine, guidelines for, 248
Diet
  in abdominal pain, 48, 49
  in angina, 54
  in ankle swelling, 58
  in arthritis, 63, 64
  in broken bones, 75
  in cancer, 80
  in congestive heart failure, 85
  in constipation, 89, 90
  in coronary artery disease, 54
  in cough, 95
  in dementia, 100
  in diabetes, 105
  in diarrhea, 110, 111
  in falls, 114
  in headache, 122
  in heart attack, 127
  in high blood pressure, 131
  in kidney failure, 133, 135, 136
  in movement disorders, 140
  in muscle or bone pain, 144
  in nausea and vomiting, 148-149
  in pressure ulcers, 158
  in psychiatric disorders, 163
  in rash, 168
  in sample care plan, 34, 36
  in seizures, 140
  in sensory impairments, 172
  in shortness of breath, 176
  in sleep problems, 152
  in stroke, 181
  in urinary incontinence, 70
  in urinary tract infections, 71
  in weakness or numbness, 185
Dietary fiber supplements, for constipation, 88
Digoxin
  for ankle swelling, 57
  for congestive heart failure, 84
  guidelines for, 248
Dilacor, guidelines for, 248
Dilantin, guidelines for, 248; *see also* Phenytoin
Dilaudid, guidelines for, 248; *see also* Hydromorphone
Diltiazem
  for angina, 53
  guidelines for, 248
  for heart attack, 126
  for high blood pressure, 130
Diphenhydramine
  guidelines for, 248
  for sleep problems, 151
Diphenoxylate, for diarrhea, 109
Diphenoxylate/atropine, guidelines for, 249
Dipyridamole, guidelines for, 249
Disalcid, guidelines for, 249
Disopyramide, guidelines for, 249
Ditropan, guidelines for, 249; *see also* Oxybutynin
Diuretics
  for ankle swelling, 57, 61
for congestive heart failure, 84
  for cough, 94
  guidelines for, 249
  for high blood pressure, 130
  hot weather and, 118
  for kidney failure, 135, 136
  for shortness of breath, 175
Divalproex, guidelines for, 249
Docusate calcium, guidelines for, 249
Donnatal, guidelines for, 249; *see also* Phenobarbital
Doxazosin
  for high blood pressure, 131
  for urinary incontinence, 67
Doxepin, guidelines for, 249
Doxycycline, guidelines for, 249
Doxylamine succinate, for sleep problems, 151
Dressings
  how to change, 159
  for pressure ulcers, 155, 156
Drug-diet interactions, 197-198
Drug-food interactions, 197
Drug interactions, 197-198
Dry skin, rash from, 166, 169
Duragesic; *see also* Fentanyl
  guidelines for, 249
  in skin patch, 214
Duricef, guidelines for, 250
Dyazide, guidelines for, 250; *see also* Triamterene/hydrochlorothiazide
DynaCirc, guidelines for, 250
Dynapen, guidelines for, 250

E
Ear medications, 171, 217-219
Ear wax removal, 217-219
Echothiophate, guidelines for, 250

Edema, of ankle, 56-61
Effexor, guidelines for, 250
Elavil, guidelines for, 250
Eldepryl, guidelines for, 250
Elder services agency, as
　resource for help, 23
Elderly
　characteristics of, 6
　specializing in, 8
Electric beds, for pressure
　ulcers, 156
Electrolyte replacement solu-
　tions, for diarrhea, 109
Elevation of legs, ankle
　swelling and, 61
Elixophyllin, guidelines for,
　250
Emotional aspects
　of cancer, 77, 81
　of dementia, 99, 101
　of falls, 113
　of heart attack, 126
　of pressure ulcers, 154-155
　of sensory impairments, 170
　of sleep problems, 150, 151
Emotional disorders, 160-164
Emphysema, 175, 177
Employees; see Staff
Enalapril
　for angina, 53
　guidelines for, 250
　for heart attack, 125
　for high blood pressure, 130
Encainide, guidelines for, 250
Enemas, 223-224
　for constipation, 89
Enkaid, guidelines for, 250
Enoxacin, guidelines for, 250
Ephedrine, guidelines for, 250
Epilepsy, after stroke, 180
Epileptic seizures, 137-141
Epinephrine
　guidelines for, 250
　in inhalers, 221

Ergostat; see Ergot
Ergot, for headache, 122
Erythromycin
　for cough, 94
　guidelines for, 251
Eserine, guidelines for, 251
Esgic-Plus, for headache, 122
Essential tremor, 137, 138, 139
Estazolam, guidelines for, 251
Estrace; see Estradiol
Estradiol
　guidelines for, 251
　for urinary incontinence, 67
Estrogens, for urinary inconti-
　nence, 67
Etodolac, guidelines for, 251
Euthroid, guidelines for, 251
Exercise
　angina and, 55
　ankle swelling and, 61
　arthritis and, 64
　cancer and, 82
　congestive heart failure and,
　　86
　diabetes and, 107
　fever and chills and, 119
　heart attack and, 126, 128
　high blood pressure and,
　　132
　movement disorders and,
　　141
　seizures and, 141
　shortness of breath and, 177
　stroke and, 182
Eye medications, 171, 214-217
　over-the-counter, 232
Eyesight disorders, 170-173

F

Falls, 112-115
Family members, as resource
　for help, 23
Famotidine
　for abdominal pain, 47

guidelines for, 251
Famvir, guidelines for, 251
Fecal impaction, diarrhea
　from, 111
Federal regulations for licens-
　ing, 18-19
Feet, numbness of, in diabetes,
　104
Feldene, guidelines for, 251
Felodipine, guidelines for, 251
Fentanyl
　for abdominal pain, 47
　guidelines for, 251
Ferrous sulfate, drug interac-
　tions with, 197
Fever, 116-119
Fiber supplements, for consti-
　pation, 88
Films, for pressure ulcers, 155,
　156
Finasteride
　guidelines for, 251
　for urinary incontinence, 68
Fioricet, for headache, 122
Fiorinal
　guidelines for, 251
　for headache, 122
Flavoxate
　guidelines for, 251
　for urinary incontinence, 67
Flecainide, guidelines for, 251
Flexeril, guidelines for, 252
Floxin, guidelines for, 252
Fluids
　in constipation, 89, 90
　sleep problems and, 153
　urinary incontinence and,
　　70, 71
Flunisolide, for cough, 94
Fluorometholone, guidelines
　for, 252
Fluoxetine
　guidelines for, 252

for psychiatric disorders, 161

Fluphenazine, guidelines for, 252

Flurazepam, guidelines for, 252

Flurbiprofen, guidelines for, 252

Flurbiprofen sodium, guidelines for, 252

Flurisolide, in inhalers, 222

Fluvastatin, guidelines for, 252

FML, guidelines for, 252

Foam mattresses, for pressure ulcers, 156

Foams, for pressure ulcers, 155, 157

Food poisoning, diarrhea from, 108-111

Foods; see also Diet
diarrhea from, 108-111
headache from, 123
for nausea and vomiting, 148-149

Forms
interfacility transfer, 40
medication administration, 196
medication record, 203
medication self-administration ability, 37
physician communication, 38

Foscavir, guidelines for, 252

Fosinopril, guidelines for, 252

Fractures, 72-76

Functional incontinence, 66

Fungal infection, rash and, 166, 167

Furosemide
for ankle swelling, 57
for congestive heart failure, 84
for cough, 94

guidelines for, 252
for kidney failure, 135
for shortness of breath, 175

G

Ganciclovir, guidelines for, 252

Gantrisin, guidelines for, 252

Garamycin, guidelines for, 253

Gauze dressings, for pressure ulcers, 155, 156

Gemfibrozil, guidelines for, 253

Gentamycin, guidelines for, 253

Geocillin, guidelines for, 253

Geopen, guidelines for, 253

Glaucoma, eye medications for, 215

Glipizide
for diabetes, 103
guidelines for, 253

Glucophage, guidelines for, 253; see also Metformin

Glucose monitoring in diabetes, 104

Glucotrol, guidelines for, 253

Glucotrol; see Glipizide

Glyburide
for diabetes, 103
guidelines for, 253

Glynase; see Glyburide

Gout, 60, 61

Government regulations for licensing, 18-19

Griseofulvin, for rash, 167

Guaifenesin, for cough, 94

Guanfacine
guidelines for, 253
for high blood pressure, 131

Guiafenesin, guidelines for, 253

H

H-2 blockers, guidelines for, 253

Halazepam, guidelines for, 253

Halcion, guidelines for, 253; see also Triazolam

Haldol, guidelines for, 254; see also Haloperidol

Haloperidol
for dementia, 99
guidelines for, 254
for psychiatric disorders, 162

Handwashing, medication administration and, 206-207

Headache, 120-123

Health status checklist, initial, 28-29

Hearing aids, 172-173

Hearing disorders, 170-173

Heart
congestive heart failure and, 83-86
high blood pressure and, 129-132

Heart attack, 52, 55, 124-128

Heart disease, 51-55

Heartburn, medication for, 47

Heat application, for muscle or bone pain, 144-145

Heat exhaustion, fever and chills and, 117

Heatstroke, fever and chills and, 117

Herplex, guidelines for, 254

High blood pressure, 129-132
weakness or numbness and, 184

Hismanal, guidelines for, 254

HMS, guidelines for, 254

Homatropine, guidelines for, 254

Home health agencies, as resource for help, 20-21

Honesty of staff, 12
Hospice programs
  for cancer, 77, 80
  as resource for help, 21
Hot weather, fever and chills and, 117, 118
Humidifiers, 220
Humorsol, guidelines for, 254
Hydralazine
  for angina, 53
  for ankle swelling, 57
  for congestive heart failure, 84
  guidelines for, 254
  for heart attack, 125
  for high blood pressure, 130
Hydrochlorothiazide
  for ankle swelling, 57
  for congestive heart failure, 84
  for cough, 94
  guidelines for, 254
  for high blood pressure, 130
  for kidney failure, 135
  for shortness of breath, 175
Hydrocodone
  for arthritis, 62
  for broken bones, 74
  guidelines for, 254
  for headache, 121
  for muscle or bone pain, 143
Hydrocolloid dressings, for pressure ulcers, 155, 156-157
Hydrocortisone
  guidelines for, 254
  for rash, 167
Hydrodiuril, guidelines for, 254
Hydrogels, for pressure ulcers, 155, 156-157
Hydromorphone
  for abdominal pain, 47
  guidelines for, 254

Hydroxychloroquine, for arthritis, 62
Hydroxyzine, guidelines for, 254
Hygroton, guidelines for, 255
Hyoscine, guidelines for, 255
Hyoscyamine, for abdominal pain, 47
Hypertension, 129-132
Hypoglycemic drugs, for diabetes, 103
Hytrin, guidelines for, 255; *see also* Terazocin

I

Ibuprofen
  for arthritis, 62
  for broken bones, 74
  for cancer, 79
  for fever and chills, 117
  guidelines for, 255
  for headache, 121
  for muscle or bone pain, 143
Ice; *see* Cold application
Idoxuridine, guidelines for, 255
Imipramine
  guidelines for, 255
  for urinary incontinence, 67
Imitrex; *see* Sumatriptan
Imodium, guidelines for, 255; *see also* Loperamide
Incontinence, urinary, 65-71
  rash from, 168, 169
Indapamide, guidelines for, 255
Inderal, guidelines for, 255; *see also* Propranolol
Indocin, guidelines for, 255; *see also* Indomethacin
Indomethacin
  for arthritis, 62
  for headache, 121

  for muscle or bone pain, 143
Infection
  ankle swelling and, 56
  arthritis and, 60
  cough and, 93
  diarrhea from, 108
  fever and chills and, 116
  of pressure ulcers, 154, 156
  rash and, 165-169
Inhalers, 220-222
Initial resident evaluation, 26-29
Injuries from falls, 112-115
Insulin, for diabetes, 104, 106
Interfacility transfer form, 40
Ipratropium
  for cough, 94
  guidelines for, 255
  in inhalers, 221
  for shortness of breath, 175
Isoptin, guidelines for, 255; *see also* Verapamil
Isordil; *see* Isosorbide dinitrate
Isosorbide dinitrate
  for angina, 53
  guidelines for, 255
  for heart attack, 125
Isradipine, guidelines for, 255

K

K-Dur, guidelines for, 256
K-Tab, guidelines for, 256
Kaolin, for diarrhea, 109
Kaon, guidelines for, 256
Kaopectate; *see* Kaolin
KCL, guidelines for, 256
Keflex, guidelines for, 256; *see also* Cephalexin
Ketoprofen, guidelines for, 256
Ketorolac, guidelines for, 256
Kidney failure, 133-136
Kidney transplantation, 135
Klonopin, guidelines for, 256

L

Labeling of medications, 198-200

Labetalol, guidelines for, 256

Lacrisert, guidelines for, 256

Lactulose, guidelines for, 256

Lanoxin, guidelines for, 256

Lasix, guidelines for, 256; *see also* Furosemide

Laws, regulating residential care facilities, 9-11

Laxatives
  for constipation, 89
  over-the-counter, 232-233

Leg elevation, ankle swelling and, 61

Lescol, guidelines for, 256

Levatol, guidelines for, 256

Level of activity; *see* Activity level

Level of care, moving to higher
  dementia and, 101
  falls and, 115
  interfacility transfer form for, 40
  outside of RCF, 39-41
  for pressure ulcers, 156, 159
  understanding need for, 25

Levobunolol, guidelines for, 256

Levocabastine, guidelines for, 256

Levodopa
  guidelines for, 256
  for movement disorders, 139
  for sleep problems, 151

Levothyroxine, guidelines for, 257

Librium, guidelines for, 257

Lice, over-the-counter medications for, 233

Licensed care nursing, 5

Licensing, 18-19

Limitations of residential care facilities, 9-11

Lincomycin, guidelines for, 257

Lioresal, guidelines for, 257

Liotrix, guidelines for, 257

Liquid medications, 209-210

Lisinopril
  for angina, 53
  guidelines for, 257
  for heart attack, 125
  for high blood pressure, 130

Lithium
  guidelines for, 257
  for psychiatric disorders, 162

Livostin, guidelines for, 257

Lodine, guidelines for, 257

Lomefloxacin, guidelines for, 257

Lomotil, guidelines for, 257; *see also* Diphenoxylate

Loperamide
  for diarrhea, 109
  guidelines for, 257

Lopid, guidelines for, 258

Lopressor, guidelines for, 257; *see also* Metoprolol

Lorazepam
  for dementia, 99
  guidelines for, 258
  for psychiatric disorders, 162

Lorelco, guidelines for, 258

Lortab, guidelines for, 258

Losartan
  for angina, 53
  for heart attack, 125-126
  for high blood pressure, 130

Lotensin, guidelines for, 258

Lovastatin, guidelines for, 258

Loxapine, guidelines for, 258

Loxitane, guidelines for, 258

Lozenges, 208-209

Lozol, guidelines for, 258

Ludiomil, guidelines for, 258

M

Maalox; *see* Magnesium/aluminum hydroxide

Magaldrate, guidelines for, 258

Magnesium/aluminum hydroxide, for abdominal pain, 47

Magnesium hydroxide, guidelines for, 258

Magnesium oxide, guidelines for, 258

Magnesium trilisate, guidelines for, 258

Malpractice, pressure ulcers and, 154, 157

Mania, 160

MAO inhibitors, diet and, 163

Mattresses, for pressure ulcers, 156

Maxaquin, guidelines for, 258

Maxzide, guidelines for, 258

MDIs; *see* Metered-dose inhalers

Meclizine, guidelines for, 258

Medical information, sample care plan and, 34, 36

Medication Quick Reference, 229-276

Medications
  ability to self-administer, 37
  administration form for "as needed," 196
  administration routes for, 208-225
    buccal, 212
    in ears, 217-219
    in eyes, 214-217
    nasal, 219-222
    oral, 208-212
    rectal, 222-224
    sublingual, 212

topical, 224-225
transdermal, 212-214
vaginal, 224
drug interactions and, 197-198
falls from, 113
guidelines for administering, 191-192
labeling of, 198-200
preparation of, 204-206
records form for, 203
refusal of, 206
sample schedule for, 194
scheduling of, 201-203
side effects of, 195
headache as, 121
Medicine cup, 212
Mellaril, guidelines for, 258; see also Thioridazine
Memory loss, dementia and, 97-101
Mental disorders, 160-164
Mentally disabled, characteristics of, 7
Meperidine, guidelines for, 258
Metaproterenol, guidelines for, 259
Metered-dose inhalers, 220-222
Metformin
for diabetes, 103
diarrhea and, 111
guidelines for, 259
Methocarbamol, guidelines for, 259
Methotrexate, for arthritis, 62
Methylcellulose, guidelines for, 259
Methylda, for high blood pressure, 131
Methyldopa, guidelines for, 259

Methylphenidate, guidelines for, 259
Metoclopramide, guidelines for, 259
Metoprolol, guidelines for, 259
Metoprolol
for angina, 53
for heart attack, 126
for high blood pressure, 130
Mevacor, guidelines for, 259
Mexiletine, guidelines for, 259
Micatin, guidelines for, 259
Miconazole, guidelines for, 259
Micro-K, guidelines for, 259
Micronase, guidelines for, 259
Migraine headache, 120-121
drugs for, 122
Milk, diarrhea from, 108, 111
Milk of magnesia, for constipation, 89
Minipres; see Prazocin
Minocin, guidelines for, 260
Misoprostol, guidelines for, 260
Missed medication, 225-226
Moban, guidelines for, 260
Molindone, guidelines for, 260
Monistat, guidelines for, 260
Monopril, guidelines for, 260
Morphine
for abdominal pain, 47
for cancer, 79
guidelines for, 260
Mortar and pestle, 210-211
Motrin, guidelines for, 260; see also Ibuprofen
Movement disorders, 137-141
MS Contin, guidelines for, 260; see also Morphine

Multiple-dose inhalers, 220-222
Multiple infarction dementia, 97
Mupirocin, guidelines for, 260
Muscle pain, 142-145
Muscular weakness, 183-186
Mycostatin; see Nystatin
Mylanta; see Magnesium/aluminum hydroxide
Myocardial infarction, 124-128
Mysoline, guidelines for, 260

N
Nabumetone, guidelines for, 260
Nadolol, guidelines for, 260
Nafcillin, guidelines for, 260
Naphazoline, guidelines for, 260
Naprosyn, guidelines for, 260; see also Naproxen
Naproxen
for arthritis, 62
guidelines for, 260
for headache, 121
for muscle or bone pain, 143
Narcotics
for abdominal pain, 47
for arthritis, 62
for cancer, 79
for cough, 96
guidelines for, 261
for headache, 121
for muscle or bone pain, 143
Nasal medications, 219-222
Nausea, 146-149
Navane, guidelines for, 261; see also Thiothixene
Nebulizers, 220
Nefazodone, guidelines for, 261
Neo-Synephrine, guidelines for, 261

Neomycin, guidelines for, 261

Neosporin; *see* Antibiotics

Nerve transmitter blocking drugs, for urinary incontinence, 67

Nerves, numbness in, 183-186

Nicardipine, guidelines for, 261

Nicotine, in skin patch, 214

Nifedepine, for high blood pressure, 130

Nifedipine
for angina, 53
guidelines for, 261
for heart attack, 126

Nitrates
for angina, 53
for heart attack, 125

Nitro-Dur, guidelines for, 261

NitroBid, guidelines for, 261

Nitrodisc, guidelines for, 261

Nitroglycerin
for angina, 53
headache from, 121
for heart attack, 125
in skin patch, 214

Nitroglycerine, guidelines for, 261

Nizatidine, guidelines for, 261

Noctec, guidelines for, 262

Nolvadex, guidelines for, 262

Nonsteroidal anti-inflammatory drugs
for arthritis, 62
for broken bones, 74
guidelines for, 262
for headache, 121
for muscle or bone pain, 143

Norflox; *see* Norfloxacin

Norfloxacin
guidelines for, 262
for urinary incontinence, 68

Normodyne, guidelines for, 262

Noroxin, guidelines for, 262

Norpace, guidelines for, 262

Norpramin, guidelines for, 262

Nortriptyline
guidelines for, 262
for psychiatric disorders, 161

Nose medications, 219-222

NPH insulin, for diabetes, 104

NSAIDs; *see* Nonsteroidal anti-inflammatory drugs

Numbness, 183-186

Nutrition; *see also* Diet
in cancer, 81
nausea and vomiting and, 146

Nystatin, for rash, 167

Nytol; *see* Diphenhydramine

O

Ocufen, guidelines for, 263

Ocupress, guidelines for, 263

Ocusert-Pilo, guidelines for, 263

Ofloxacin, guidelines for, 263

Omeprazole
for abdominal pain, 47
guidelines for, 263

Open fracture, 73

Ophthalmics, 214-217

Oral medications, 208-212

Oramorph-SR; *see* Morphine

Orfloxacin, guidelines for, 263

Orientation of employees, 14-15

Orinase, guidelines for, 263

Orudis, guidelines for, 263

Osteoarthritis, 60

Osteoporosis, broken bones from, 72

Ostomy, cancer and, 81

OTC drugs; *see* Over-the-counter drugs

Otics, 217-219

Over-the-counter drugs
labeling of, 199, 200
in Medication Quick Reference, 231-233

Overflow incontinence, 66

Oxacillin, guidelines for, 263

Oxaprozin, guidelines for, 263

Oxazepam
for dementia, 99
for psychiatric disorders, 162

Oxybutynin
guidelines for, 263
for urinary incontinence, 67

Oxycodone, guidelines for, 263

Oxymetazoline, guidelines for, 263

Oxytriphylline, guidelines for, 263

P

Pain medications, over-the-counter, 232

Pamelor, guidelines for, 263; *see also* Nortriptyline

Pancrelipase, guidelines for, 263

Panic disorders, 160

Parafon forte, guidelines for, 263

Parkinson's disease, movement disorders in, 137-141

Parlodel, guidelines for, 264; *see also* Pergolide

Paroxetine, guidelines for, 264

Patient's bill of rights, 16-17

Paxil, guidelines for, 264

Paxipam, guidelines for, 264

Penetrex, guidelines for, 264

Penicillin G, guidelines for, 264

Pentazocine, guidelines for, 264

Pentoxifylline, guidelines for, 264

Pepcid, guidelines for, 264; *see also* Famotidine

Percocet, guidelines for, 264

Pergolide, for movement disorders, 139

Periactin, guidelines for, 264

Peritoneal dialysis, 134

Perphenazine, guidelines for, 264

Persantine, guidelines for, 264

Pharmacy, working with, 191-192

Phenazopyridine, guidelines for, 264

Phenergan, guidelines for, 264

Phenobarbital
for abdominal pain, 47
guidelines for, 264
for seizures, 139

Phenylephrine, guidelines for, 265

Phenylpropanolamine, guidelines for, 265

Phenytoin
guidelines for, 265
for seizures, 139

Phlegm, cough and, 92

Phospholine iodide, guidelines for, 265

Phrenilin, for headache, 122

Physically disabled, characteristics of, 7-8

Physician communication form, 38

Physostigmine, guidelines for, 265

Pilocarpine
for eye disorders, 171
guidelines for, 265

Pinched nerve, 186

Pindolol, guidelines for, 265

Piroxicam, guidelines for, 265

Plaquenil; *see* Hydroxychloroquine

Plendil, guidelines for, 265

Pneumonia, cough and, 93

Polycillin, guidelines for, 265

Polymyxin B, guidelines for, 265

Polypharmacy, 226-227

Postictal state, 138

Pramoxine, guidelines for, 265

Pravachol, guidelines for, 265

Prazocin
for high blood pressure, 131
for urinary incontinence, 67

Prednisone
for arthritis, 62
for cough, 94
guidelines for, 265
for kidney failure, 135
for shortness of breath, 175

Premarin, guidelines for, 266; *see also* Conjugated estrogen

Pressure reducing devices, for pressure ulcers, 156

Pressure ulcers, 154-159

Prevacid, guidelines for, 266

Prilosec, guidelines for, 266; *see also* Omeprazole

Primidone, guidelines for, 266

Prinivil, guidelines for, 266; *see also* Lisinopril

PRN medications, 193-195
sample administration form for, 196
scheduling of, 202

Probanthine, guidelines for, 266; *see also* Propantheline

Probenecid
for arthritis, 62
guidelines for, 266

Probucol, guidelines for, 266

Procainamide, guidelines for, 266

Procardia, guidelines for, 266; *see also* Nifedipine

Prochlorperazine
for cancer, 79
guidelines for, 266
for nausea and vomiting, 147

Profenal, guidelines for, 266

Prolixin, guidelines for, 266

Promazine, guidelines for, 266

Promethazine, guidelines for, 266

Pronestyl, guidelines for, 266

Propafenone, guidelines for, 266

Propantheline
guidelines for, 267
for urinary incontinence, 67

Propoxyphene, guidelines for, 267

Propranolol
for angina, 53
guidelines for, 267
for heart attack, 126

Proscar, guidelines for, 267; *see also* Finasteride

ProSom, guidelines for, 267

Prostaphlin, guidelines for, 267

Prostate shrinking drugs, for urinary incontinence, 68

Proventil, guidelines for, 267; *see also* Albuterol

Prozac, guidelines for, 267; *see also* Fluoxetine

Pseudoephedrine, guidelines for, 267

Psychiatric disorders, 160-164

Psychosis, 161

Punch cards, 200, 205

Pus
cough and, 92
rash and, 165

Pyridium, guidelines for, 267

Q

Questran, guidelines for, 267
Quinapril, guidelines for, 267
Quinidex, guidelines for, 267
Quinidine, guidelines for, 267
Quinine, guidelines for, 267

R

Ramipril, guidelines for, 268
Ranitidine
   for abdominal pain, 47
   guidelines for, 268
Rash, 165-169
RCFs; *see* Residential care
   facilities
Records; *see also* Forms
   admission, 27
   keeping current, 32-39
Rectal medications, 222-224
Reglan, guidelines for, 268
Regular insulin, for diabetes,
   104
Regulations for residential care
   facilities, 9-11
Rehabilitation, after stroke,
   180-181
Relafen, guidelines for, 268
Religious organizations, as
   resource for help, 21-22
Replacement therapy, 191,
   192
Resident needs, more than
   can be provided, 39-41
Resident review process, 39
Residential care facilities, 3-23
   growing need for, 3-4
   other terms used for, 3
   resources for, 19-23
   responsibilities and limita-
      tions of, 8-12
   role of, 4-6
   specializing in elderly and, 8

staffing for, 12-19
types of residents in, 6-8
Residents
   types of, 6-8
   understanding needs of, 25-
      26
Resources, 18-23
Respiration, shortness of
   breath and, 175-177
Responsibilities of residential
   care facilities, 9-11
Restoril, guidelines for, 268;
      see also Temazepam
Review process, 228-229
Rheumatoid arthritis, 60, 61
Rib fracture, 76
Rights of patients, 16-17
Riopan; *see* Magnesium/
   aluminum hydroxide
Ritalin, guidelines for, 268
Robaxin, guidelines for, 268
Robitussin; *see* Guaifenesin
Rules of conduct, 12-13
Rythmol, guidelines for, 268

S

Safety, 10-11
Salsalate, guidelines for, 268
Salt
   congestive heart failure and,
      84, 85
   kidney failure and, 135
Sansert; *see* Ergot
Scabies
   over-the-counter medica-
      tions for, 233
   skin rash and, 169
Scheduling of medication use,
   201-203
`sample, 194
Schizophrenia, 160, 161
Scopolamine
   for abdominal pain, 47
   guidelines for, 268

in skin patch, 214
Seaweed dressings, for pressure
   ulcers, 155, 157
Sectral, guidelines for, 268
Security, 10-11
Sedatives
   for dementia, 99
   for headache, 122
Seizures, 137-141
   after stroke, 180
Seldane, guidelines for, 268
Selegiline, guidelines for, 268
Sensory impairments, 170-173
Septra, guidelines for, 269;
      see also Trimethoprim/
         sulfamethoxazole
Serax; *see* Oxazepam
Sertraline
   guidelines for, 269
   for psychiatric disorders, 161
Serzone, guidelines for, 269
Shingles, 168-169
Shortness of breath, 174-177
Shunts, in kidney dialysis, 133-
   134
Side effects of medications,
   195, 228
Silent heart attack, 125
Simethicone, guidelines for,
   269
Simvastatin, guidelines for, 269
Sinemet, guidelines for, 269;
      see also Levodopa
Sinequan, guidelines for, 269
Skin cancer, 79
Skin infection; *see also*
   Infection
      ankle swelling and, 57
Skin moisturizers, for rash, 167
Skin patches, 212-214
Skin rash, 165-169
Skin ulcers, 154-159
Sleep apnea, headache from,
   123

Sleep problems, 150-153
Sleeping pills, 151, 153
Slipped disk, pinched nerve and, 186
Slo-bid, guidelines for, 269
Smell disorders, 170-173
Smoking, shortness of breath and, 175, 177
Social groups, as resource for help, 22
Social Security Act, licensing and, 18
Social services
    as resource for help, 20
    sample care plan and, 33-34, 35
Sodium phosphate, guidelines for, 269
Sodium sulfacetamide, guidelines for, 269
Sominex; *see* Diphenhydramine
Sorbitrate, guidelines for, 269
Sparine, guidelines for, 269
Spectrobid, guidelines for, 269
Splitting tablets, 209
Sputum, cough and, 92
Stable angina, 52
Staff, 11-17; *see also* Caregivers
State laws
    for licensing, 19
    on medication administration, 190
    on medication labeling, 198-199
Steroids
    for arthritis, 62
    for cough, 94
    for rash, 167
    for shortness of breath, 175
Stimulant laxatives, for constipation, 89
Stomach inflammation, medication for, 47

Stomach pain; *see* Abdominal pain
Stomach ulcer
    description and causes of, 49
    medication for, 47
Stool softeners
    for constipation, 88
    diarrhea from, 108
Stools
    arthritis medication and, 61
    constipation and, 87-91
    diarrhea and, 108-111
    muscle or bone pain and, 143
Storage of medications, 204
Stress incontinence, 66
Stroke, 178-182
    weakness or numbness and, 183, 184, 186
Sublingual medications, 212, 213
Sucralfate
    for abdominal pain, 47
    guidelines for, 269
Sudafed, guidelines for, 270
Sugar diabetes; *see* Diabetes
Suicide, 161
Sulamyd, guidelines for, 270
Sulfisoxazole, guidelines for, 270
Sumatriptan, for headache, 122
Suppositories
    rectal, 222-224
    vaginal, 224
Suprax, guidelines for, 270
Suprofen, guidelines for, 270
Sustained-release medications, 210
Swallowing difficulties, diet in, 185, 186
Sweating, drug side effects and, 118

Symmetrel, guidelines for, 270
Synagogues, as resource for help, 21-22
Synthroid, guidelines for, 270

T
Tablets, 208
Tacrine, for dementia, 98
Tagamet, guidelines for, 270; *see also* Cimetidine
Talwin, guidelines for, 270
Tambocor, guidelines for, 270
Tamoxifen, guidelines for, 270
Tardive dyskinesia, 137, 138
Taste disorders, 170-173
Tegopen, guidelines for, 270
Tegretol, guidelines for, 270; *see also* Carbamazepine
Temazepam
    guidelines for, 271
    for sleep problems, 151
Temperature, body; *see* Body temperature
Tenes; *see* Guanfacine
Tenex, guidelines for, 271
Tenormin, guidelines for, 271; *see also* Atenolol
Tension headache, 120
Terazocin
    guidelines for, 271
    for high blood pressure, 131
    for urinary incontinence, 67
Terfenadine, guidelines for, 271
Tessalon perles; *see* Benzonatate
Tetracycline
    for cough, 94
    drug interactions with, 197
    guidelines for, 271
Tetrahydrozoline, guidelines for, 271
Theo-Dur, guidelines for, 271

Theophylline, guidelines for, 271

Thioridazine
  for dementia, 99
  guidelines for, 271
  for psychiatric disorders, 162

Thiothixene
  guidelines for, 271
  for psychiatric disorders, 162

Thorazine, guidelines for, 271

Thyroid replacement therapy, 192

Ticlid, guidelines for, 271

Tigan, guidelines for, 271;
    see also
    Trimethobenzamide

Time-release medications, 210

Timolol
  for eye disorders, 171
  guidelines for, 272

Timoptic, guidelines for, 272;
    see also Timolol

Tindal, guidelines for, 272

Titrolac; *see* Calcium carbonate

Tobramycin, guidelines for, 272

Tocainide, guidelines for, 272

Tofranil, guidelines for, 272;
    see also Imipramine

Tolazamide
  for diabetes, 103
  guidelines for, 272

Tolbutamide, guidelines for, 272

Tolectin, guidelines for, 272

Tolinase, guidelines for, 272;
    see also Tolazamide

Tolmetin, guidelines for, 272

Tonocard, guidelines for, 272

Topical medications, 224-225

Toprol; *see* Metaprolol

Toradol, guidelines for, 272

Training of employees, 14-15

Tramadol, guidelines for, 272

Tramcinolone, in inhalers, 221-222

Transdermal medications, 212-214

Tranxene, guidelines for, 272

Trazodone, guidelines for, 272

Tremor, 137-141

Trental, guidelines for, 272

Triamcinolone
  for cough, 94
  for rash, 167

Triamterene/hydrochlorothiazide
  for ankle swelling, 57
  for congestive heart failure, 84
  for cough, 94
  guidelines for, 273
  for high blood pressure, 130
  for kidney failure, 135
  for shortness of breath, 175

Triavil, guidelines for, 273

Triazolam
  guidelines for, 273
  for sleep problems, 151

Tricyclic antidepressants, guidelines for, 273

Trifluridine, guidelines for, 273

Trihexyphenidyl, guidelines for, 273

Trilafon, guidelines for, 273

Trimethobenzamide
  for cancer, 79
  guidelines for, 273
  for nausea and vomiting, 147

Trimethoprim/sulfamethoxazole
  for cough, 94
  guidelines for, 273
  for urinary incontinence, 68

Troches, 208-209

Tuberculosis

cough and, 93
routine testing for, 96

Tums; *see* Calcium carbonate

Tylenol; *see* Acetaminophen

Tylenol with codeine, guidelines for, 273

U

Ulcer
  description and causes of, 49
  pressure, 154-159

Ultracef, guidelines for, 273

Ultram, guidelines for, 273

Unipen, guidelines for, 274

Uniphyl, guidelines for, 274

Unisom; *see* Doxylamine succinate

Unlicensed facilities, government regulations and, 19

Unstable angina, 52

Urecholine, guidelines for, 274

Urge incontinence, 66

Urinary catheterization, incontinence and, 71

Urinary frequency, 65

Urinary incontinence, 65-71
  hot weather and, 118
  rash from, 168, 169

Urinary retention, 65, 70-71

Urinary tract infections, diet and, 71

Urispas, guidelines for, 274;
    see also Flavoxate

Urocholine; *see* Bethanechol

V

Vaginal medications, 224

Valium, guidelines for, 274;
    see also Diazepam

Valproic acid, guidelines for, 274

Vanceril, for shortness of breath, 175; *see also* Beclomethasone

Vancocin, guidelines for, 274

Vancomycin, guidelines for, 274

Vantin, guidelines for, 274

Vaporizers, 220

Variant angina, 52

Vascor, guidelines for, 274

Vasodilators
  for angina, 53
  for ankle swelling, 57
  for congestive heart failure, 84
  for heart attack, 125-126
  for high blood pressure, 130

Vasotec, guidelines for, 274; see also Enalapril

Velosef, guidelines for, 274

Venlafaxine, guidelines for, 274

Ventolin, guidelines for, 275; see also Albuterol

Verapamil
  for angina, 53
  guidelines for, 275
  for heart attack, 126
  for high blood pressure, 130

Vibramycin, guidelines for, 275

Vicodin, guidelines for, 275; see also Hydrocodone

Vira-A, guidelines for, 275

Viral infections, rash and, 167, 168-169

Viroptic, guidelines for, 275

Vision disorders, 170-173

Visken, guidelines for, 275

Vistaril, guidelines for, 275

Voltaren, guidelines for, 275

Vomiting, 146-149

W

Warfarin, guidelines for, 275

Water mattresses, for pressure ulcers, 156

Water pills; see Diuretics

Weakness, 183-186

Wellbutrin, guidelines for, 275

Wet gauze dressings, for pressure ulcers, 155, 156

Withdrawal headache, 121

Wrong medication/dose, 226

X

Xanax, guidelines for, 275; see also Alprazolam

Xylometazoline, guidelines for, 275

Y

Young residents, in residential care facilities, 7-8

Z

Zantac, guidelines for, 275; see also Ranitidine

Zestril, guidelines for, 276; see also Lisinopril

Zinacef, guidelines for, 276

Zithromax, guidelines for, 276

Zocor, guidelines for, 276

Zoloft, guidelines for, 276

Zolott; see Sertraline

Zolpidem
  guidelines for, 276
  for sleep problems, 151

Zovirax; see Acyclovir

Zyloprim, guidelines for, 276; see also Allopurinol